Pulling Taffy

A Year with Dementia and Other Adventures

by Tinky Weisblat

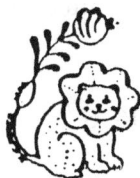

The Merry Lion Press
Hawley, Massachusetts

The Merry Lion Press
84 Middle Road
Hawley, MA 01339

Visit the book's web site at www.pullingtaffy.com for more information.

First printing 2013.

Publisher's Cataloging-in-Publication Data

Weisblat, Tinky
Pulling taffy: a year with dementia and other adventures
by Tinky Weisblat

ISBN 978-0-9742741-0-2

   1. Weisblat, Tinky. 2. Weisblat, Janice Hallett—1918-
      2011. 3. Alzheimer's disease—Patients—United States.
      4. Alzheimer's disease—Patients—United States—
      Biography. 5. Mothers and Daughters—United States.
      6. Aging parents—Care—United States.

Library of Congress Control Number: 2013900436

Printed in the United States of America.

CONTENTS

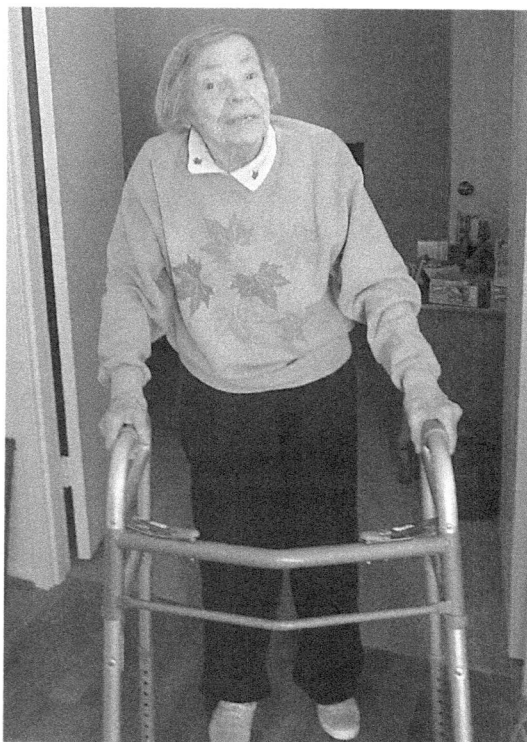

About the Illustrations

The photographs in this book are in general NOT professional. They are snapshots taken by the author and her friends, intended to add a visual element to the book. All are copyrighted (2013) by the Merry Lion Press. The cover photo was taken by R. Peter Beck.

SNAPSHOT

Tuesday, May 22: Floored

Two days ago my poor mother ended up on the floor for a while. And I was reminded of a lesson I seem to need to keep on learning.

Taffy went into her bedroom in the late morning. I heard her walker move to the window. She loves gazing at the trees and people outdoors.

Soon all was silent.

I presumed she had decided to lie down on her bed to nap. She had risen early that morning so I knew she was due for a little extra shuteye.

When I peeked in on her a few minutes later, she was perched on the sides of a cardboard box on the floor, dozing.

The whole setup looked AMAZINGLY awkward. The box holds knickknacks, albums, and framed photos for which we haven't yet found homes in our new apartment. Taffy was poised in lopsided fashion above the box's contents … and sinking fast.

I woke her and tried to get her to stand up, but she insisted that she was comfortable. "The problem is," I said, "that you won't be comfortable for long."

The box proved my point by making a little crumpling sound to indicate that it was preparing to go down for the count.

I grabbed the sides of the box and gently tipped Taffy out onto the carpeted floor so that she wouldn't fall and hurt herself.

Getting her off the floor proved more complicated. She's not at all heavy, but she was determined to stay on the floor and nap—so she resisted mightily when I tried to lift her up. I thought about pushing, crying, and screaming. Instead I bided my time.

One thing I've learned from dealing with Taffy lately is the value of waiting when things get complicated. Arguing, yelling, crying, and otherwise working myself up don't help either of us.

In 20 minutes she was delighted to have me help her up. She moved on to nap on the living-room couch, where she looked a LOT more comfortable.

Biding my time was harder late that night when she once again became determined to steer her own course.

It was one of those evenings during which she has a lot of trouble going to sleep. I peeked in at 11:30 as I was getting ready to go to bed.

She was sitting on the toilet in her pajamas, convinced that if she went back to bed someone would come in and murder her. She was extraordinarily tired so she suspected I was in cahoots with whoever it was.

I let her be for 20 minutes and then came back. I managed to move her to her bedside chair, but that was as far as she would go.

I almost left her there, but the chair is not the steadiest in the world, and I didn't want her falling off. So I took the dog for a quick walk, brushed my teeth, and then read for a little while. In another half hour she was ready to return to her bed.

Part of me felt triumphant that I had managed to get her into bed without upsetting either of us more—and part of me felt just plain exhausted.

Today we are going to the doctor for tests. I hope he will be able to figure out what is making Taffy extra confused and paranoid these days. We have already determined that her urinary-tract infections—which accelerate behavior like Sunday's—are not ordinary ones. With luck, we'll soon know what they are. With even more luck, they will be treatable.

Meanwhile, I comfort myself that I am cultivating patience, a virtue that has never been one of my strengths.

As I think about it, perching on a box near the floor is probably some kind of metaphor for the balancing act my mother and I perform every day as her dementia increases. She is suspended precariously. I try to guide her ever so gently. And we hope that nothing will collapse underneath us.

ABOUT THIS BOOK

This book is about a mother and a daughter ... and therefore about parents and children in general. It's about dementia and about death. Mostly, it's about trying to live with humor, joy, and patience.

These words may sound sentimental. They shouldn't. I pride myself on not being overly sentimental. I try to be honest, however. And the last couple of years have taught me that when push comes to shove—and it all too frequently does—we humans are sunk without humor, joy, and patience. Especially humor.

As baby boomers age, Alzheimer's disease is becoming a daily reality for many Americans. The Alzheimer's Association reports that approximately 5.2 million people in the United States suffer from the disease. More than 15 million unpaid caregivers take care of them.

Until December 2011 I was one of those caregivers.

In the years leading up to her death in that month I lived with and took care of my mother Jan. The experience was frustrating, moving, and in the end rewarding. It brought me tears. It brought me laughter as well. I hope to share the tears and especially the laughter here in *Pulling Taffy*.

The title was suggested by my friend Peter. It fit our situation to a T. Taffy was a long-standing family nickname for my mother. And the concept of a taffy pull, in which people have to work together—are in a sense stuck together—was appropriate. For several years I was yoked to my mother. Taking care of her was work, albeit sometimes sweet work.

I write for a living—mostly about food and the media—so it was only natural for me to write about my time with my mother. I kept a private journal and shared much of it online in blog form.

This book shares journal and blog entries from 2011, my last year with Taffy, as well as some retrospective essays and thoughts. The snapshot you just read is one of the entries.

When I started in January 2011 I planned to keep writing for a year. I had no idea that fate was going to round out the year and give my family closure at the end of 2011.

At first my essays provided me with a forum in which I could find a release for my frustrations in dealing with Taffy and her illness. I wrote about tears in the night (mostly mine, I am sorry to report!), the pleasure of taking bubble baths when I finally managed to get my mother into bed, and my fears about losing her if she wandered out the door alone.

My writing—and our journey together—changed in remarkable ways as the year went on.

I continued to discuss my difficulties in taking care of my mother. More and more, however, I meditated on the changes in both of our lives and explored the ways in which my mother's mode of looking at the world altered as her brain deteriorated ... and the ways in which that mode of looking at the world remained the same. I also increasingly chronicled positive aspects of my caregiving experience.

Bookstore shelves are lined with books by children who have cared for parents with dementia. Some of the books share stories of conflict and tragedy. Others offer medical advice. Most of them are touching to read.

So ... why should anyone read another book about this experience? I believe this book deserves a place on those crowded bookstore shelves for several reasons.

First of all, its journal format gives readers a sense of my mother's experiences and mine as they happened. I have cleaned up a few grammatical peccadilloes in the story's transformation from journal to book. I haven't altered events or tried to shape them into an overarching narrative. Time and fate provided the narrative. This book therefore gives readers unusual immediacy in its portrayal of life with dementia that most other books on the subject lack.

Second, I want to throw my two cents into the ring on the subject of what dementia does and doesn't do to those who suffer from it.

Several books I've read about taking care of people with Alzheimer's—most notably Barry Peterson's *Jan's Story* (2010) and Andrea Gillies's *Keeper* (2009)—dwell on the dark side of dementia. In each case the caregiver (a husband in Peterson's case, a daughter-in-law in Gillies's) sees the disease as taking away the self of the person who suffers from it.

I don't mean to pretend that Alzheimer's has no dark moments. I sympathize deeply with both of these writers, particularly Peterson, whose wife developed early-onset Alzheimer's disease in her 50s. Nevertheless, in my experience much of a person's selfhood remains as this complicated disease inhabits more and more of the brain.

Alzheimer's may erase many things about a person—memories, vocabulary, adult reasoning—but fundamentally it can't erase the human spirit. Again and again throughout the year I was struck by the ways in which my mother's essence was always with us. It is with me as I write this several months after her death.

I hope my story will encourage people who are in rough personal situations such as living with Alzheimer's disease, either as a patient or a caregiver. My mother was not extraordinary; nor am I. Our ordinariness, in fact, is the point of our story. The things that helped us get through the year and find happy moments again and again are ordinary, too. They are available to just about everyone.

As I indicated at the top of this introduction, the first was laughter. It invariably made our burdens lighter and brought us together. It was occasionally hard to find, but the search for the lighter side of our experiences always proved worthwhile.

The second was community. Time and again we reached out to family, friends, neighbors, and our church for support. Often we didn't even have to reach out. People just appeared. They brought food. They cheered us up. They visited with Taffy for a while to give me a break.

When one hits a family crisis, one (this one, at any rate) sometimes feels an impulse to pull inward and not ask for help. My experience is that if people understand what is needed (and one does have to specify sometimes), they will come through.

Our last bulwark was music. We listened to music in recordings and at concerts, sang songs together, conducted imaginary orchestras, improvised a little percussion. Music enriched our lives time and again, making us feel physically and spiritually better.

Beyond sharing these strategies, ruminating on the essence of life, and describing day-to-day dealings with dementia, this book pays tribute to my mother. Taffy lived her life with joy and love. Hers was a spirit we can all emulate.

At the end of each month of my chronicle of our year together I append an essay I wrote after her death, as well as a recipe. The recipes represent the importance of cooking and shared meals in our family life.

The essays try to round out the story told by the journal entries. A couple of these monthly "meditations" talk about practical matters that may be of interest to other patients and caregivers. One discusses the help we hired to get Taffy (and me!) through her final year. The other presents a few tips for other caregivers.

Most of the essays, however, recall portions of Taffy's life. These reminiscences link the Taffy of her final year to the woman she was for the 92 years before the book begins. The different Taffys are scattered throughout the book like pieces of a kaleidoscope. I hope the reader can use them to shift perspective and glimpse her life as a whole in all its richness and color.

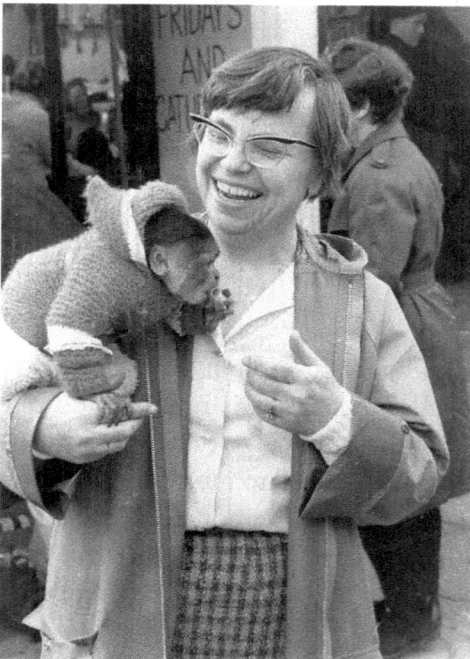

*My mother
with a friend
in 1968*

JANUARY
Beginnings

Saturday, January 1: Baby Steps

The first tears of the new year came very early on the morning of January 1, at 1:15 a.m. to be precise. They began to flow about 45 minutes after I went to bed, about five hours after Taffy did.

The tears were mine. They almost always are. I have extremely active tear ducts. Mostly I cry at movies—I can't get through *Casablanca* or *Now, Voyager* without serious tissue support—but from time to time I succumb to non-cinematic sadness when the dementia is raging, particularly in the middle of the night.

I seem to need nine hours of uninterrupted sleep to maintain my equilibrium. If I get fewer hours, I'm grumpy and/or tearful.

ANYWAY, here's what happened in the wee hours:

I awoke from a deep sleep to find my mother in the living room, fully dressed, ready to go out. She has a little trouble telling night from day in recent months, particularly after days during which she has napped a lot. Yesterday—Friday, December 31—was one of those days.

During the day on Friday Pertina, the caregiver who blessedly comes three days a week for a few hours, read with Taffy and tried to get her to do a jigsaw puzzle. I chatted with Taffy, sang a couple of songs with her, and tried to get her to go out with me or watch something fun on television. She fell asleep on both of us before we got very far.

So there she was at one this morning, ready to rock and roll.

Getting her to go back into her bed was relatively easy on this occasion. (Sometimes she's unwilling.) Getting her back into her pajamas, however, proved futile.

I fussed at her a bit. (I know fussing doesn't do much good with dementia sufferers, but I'm not at my best when awakened from sound sleep.)

In the end, however, I stopped crying, tucked her into bed with her clothes on, and wished her a happy new year. There are some battles not worth fighting, some tears not worth shedding.

She smiled as she went back to sleep.

Alas, our dog Truffle decided she desperately had to go outside a couple of hours later—a little too much New Year's Eve lasagna perhaps?—but that's another story.

Much later this morning while Taffy slept my friend Peter called to share new year's news.

He told me he is convinced I belong on television.

Of course I agree with him. I am, let's face it, vivacious, smart, and talented. There are just a couple of teensy obstacles.

I need contacts (the people, not the lenses).

And I need to get the Tinky body back into shape. The past year has been very hard on my not-so-svelte-to-start-with figure.

I have resolved (ooh, that word) to start trying to make some contacts this week. Meanwhile, I can at least eat fairly sensibly, get a small amount of exercise (since I can't leave Taffy this involves walking or dancing around the apartment), and work on getting a haircut. Make that two haircuts: the mother needs one as well.

Baby steps, baby steps....

Thursday, January 6: Someone's in the Kitchen with Tinky

Cooking with a person who suffers from dementia is like cooking with a small child. Happily, my mother can still wield a knife, more or less. But the kitchen tasks she performs must be carefully chosen as they would be for a little one. She can only think about one small task at a time. And she is easily frustrated.

Sometimes the head chef becomes a little frustrated too. Cooking with my mother helps me cultivate the art of patience—and reminds me that process is as important as product in cooking.

I am lucky that cooking is rewarding for Taffy at this stage. She longs daily to do something useful; she has been a highly useful person all her life. Yet there are now very few things she can do even vaguely efficiently.

When we cook together she still feels that she is contributing to the household. And that makes both of us happy.

Yesterday we prepared a simple Twelfth Night (okay, technically Eleventh Night) supper to share with our extended family—my brother David, his wife Leigh, and their son Michael.

I did the lioness's share of the cooking since it was a big nap day for Taffy. She helped prep the vegetables for our soup, however, and supervised the creation of a rustic apple tart.

Our vegetable beef soup was simple yet satisfying, perfect for an evening repast during National Soup Month.

I'm sharing the soup recipe at the end of this chapter since Taffy and I co-created it. In fact, it was she who taught me to make soup many years ago. Be sure to sing a final Christmas carol as you cook your soup. We did!

Fa la la la la, la la la la.

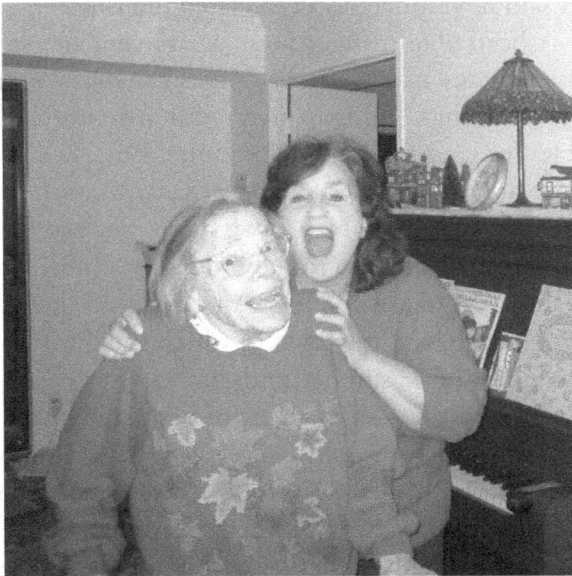

Monday, January 10: A Longing for Home

One characteristic my mother shares with many Alzheimer's patients is a desire to go "home." It has been particularly strong in recent days.

I can often distract her from it—usually with an excursion in the car, which again seems to be common. One of my blog readers, Pam, wrote these words in response to one of my essays about Taffy:

"Nearly every evening Mom would call me to say that Dad was ready for me to come and 'take him home.' Home evidently being his childhood home. I would drive over, Dad would be in coat and hat, and off we would go. We just drove around awhile and then went back to their condo where Dad always thanked me very kindly and said how much he appreciated the ride!"

I haven't been able to figure out what event or phenomenon (if any) precipitates my mother's homesickness. We are in new physical surroundings, an apartment near my brother's home in Virginia. Her longing to go home precedes the new digs, however. Wherever we are, sooner or later she is ready to go home. Telling her that she is in fact home may satisfy her—but not for long.

Sometimes her longing to be home is quite specific. On Thursday she was focused on getting back to her parents in Maplewood, New Jersey, the town in which she lived from the age of two or so until she was in her mid-20s.

I generally try to finesse the issue of her parents when she asks about them. If she is in a particularly rational frame of mind, I explain that they both died years ago. If she is not, I don't upset her by breaking the "news" of their deaths to her. Often we compromise. She talks about her parents in the present tense. I talk about them in the past tense.

While I'm sometimes frustrated by Taffy's longing for her parents I'm also fascinated by it. My mother adored her father. She was his pet, his smart girl, his "Punkins." The only time I've seen her really upset is when he died in 1966—although, being the sensible woman that she was, she mostly felt relief that his suffering was over.

Interestingly, although he didn't generally suffer from dementia, shortly before he died my grandfather (shown here) told Taffy about a delightful buggy ride he had taken that very afternoon with his long-dead father.

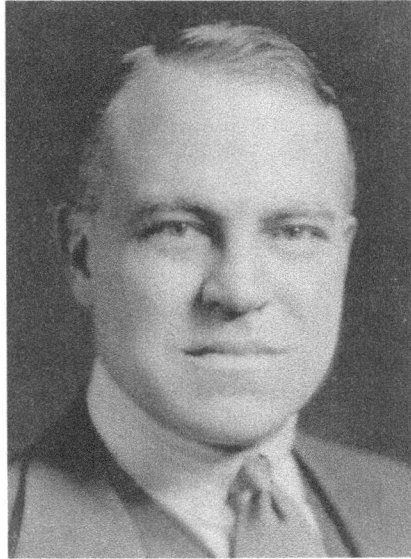

She said she had seldom seen her father happier than when he talked about this excursion.

She was attached to her mother, and she was a responsible caregiver when my grandmother suffered from dementia in her 90s. I don't recall that my mother expressed a great deal of affection toward her own mother as an adult or remembered her mother as an especially affectionate parent to Jan the child, however.

The longing for her mother at this point seems to be a generic longing for a mother—an attachment to the idea of a mother rather than an attachment to the real woman who bore Taffy, raised her, and romantically named her Janice after the heroine in the novel *Janice Meredith*.

Although my mother often talks about Maplewood and can certainly recall the houses in which she lived there better than any house she has lived in since, I think my mother's longing for home, like her longing for her mother, may be symbolic—a longing for an archetype rather than a real memory.

It seems to be a longing to feel at peace, to feel comfortable with herself, to feel safe, to feel normal.

Somewhere deep in her not-all-there brain, then, Taffy is wisely expressing a universal human longing for the wider meaning of the word "home."

A few nights ago we watched *E.T.*, a film that addresses the longing for home in many ways. Now when my mother tells me she wants to call home, I think, "E.T., phone home." She is clearly feeling a little alien in her surroundings, despite the love all around her.

So if she wants to go home, I do what I can to deflect her gently. We recite poems, sing songs, look at books of family photos, and/or hop in the car. (Sometimes I even get her to take a nap so she can lose her restlessness in actual rest and I can get a little work done.)

If all else fails I call in the family, and we all tell her we love her—and remind her that home is above all a place of love.

These strategies don't completely satisfy her. For a while, however, they make all of us feel a little more comfortable in our surroundings, a little more at home.

Thursday, January 13: A Moment of Identification

Taffy woke up this morning at 3:30 VERY confused, not knowing who or where she was and asking for her mother.

I did the best I could. Bringing the dog in to cuddle with my mother worked even better than my hugs. Within the hour she was back asleep.

As I lay back down on my own bed I thought about what this experience must be like for Taffy.

I move around a lot so at least two or three times a year I have a tiny taste of it. After a particularly vivid dream during my first night in a new place, I wake up suddenly and find that I am not in the room I expected to be in.

Within a few minutes I get my bearings and feel comfortable again—but the initial feeling of being in a strange place is quite eerie.

I believe that feeling must approach what my mother goes through almost every night.

Friday, January 14: Cookie Monster

Like many elders, my mother has lost some of her sense of taste. I don't know why this should astonish me since she has definitely lost much of her capacity for seeing, hearing, and smelling things. Losing one's taste buds, I gather, is a natural occurrence in the old.

Nevertheless, it always takes me a little by surprise when she isn't interested in foods that formerly delighted her, particularly spicy foods—curry, salsa, and so forth. Even odder, given her past, is her current passion for sweets.

My mother spent much of her life avoiding sweets. Her idea of a fancy dessert was fresh fruit.

She avoided sweets in part because she was always battling her weight. (I can relate to that!) She also avoided them, so she said, because she didn't particularly care for them.

Today she is a fiend for sweet things—particularly cookies. She will nibble vaguely at a sandwich for lunch and then request dessert when the main course is less than a quarter eaten. Clearly, she can still taste sweets if very little else.

Although Taffy's passion for sweets seems unhealthy it does give me leverage. I generally try to avoid infantilizing her. When it comes to food, however, I have no trouble treating her like a small child. I tell her that she may have dessert IF she eats most of her "real" food.

I think her desire for sweets relates to her memory issues as well as her taste buds. She frequently forgets that she has eaten recently. Yesterday an hour after breakfast she informed me that I hadn't fed her in a couple of days.

The sugar high from sweets gives her an immediate feeling of having been fed.

So I muddle along, mixing as many healthy things into her diet as I can but being sure to give her a cookie or two each day. She is no longer at all heavy, and if small things make her happy, I say, "Let her have them!"

Besides, it's hard not to see her sweet tooth as a physiological representation of much of her experience at this point in her life. As she ages and forgets things, she wants more of the sweet things the world has to offer. She has consumed nourishing soups and salads all her life. Now she is looking for the icing on the cake (and preferably a bite or two of cake as well)

Today we made buttery cookies for my cookie monster. Our hand mixer seems to have only one beater, but that didn't worry Taffy. The other beater is SOMEWHERE in the kitchen ... I think. (I have my own memory issues!)

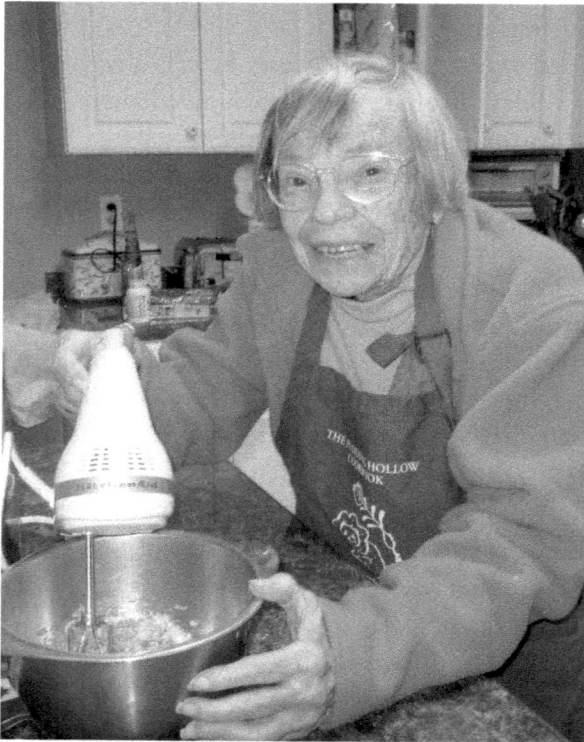

Friday, January 21: It Takes a Village

Fellow caregivers—or people who are stressed out for any reason: If you are feeling overwhelmed, reach out. Someone is almost always there to help you.

A couple of afternoons ago I was just about at the end of my tether with my mother. I was writing to deadline, and I had almost finished my article.

"Almost" can seem very far from "completely," however. It felt as though I would never take that tiny last step.

Often Taffy nods off in the afternoon, particularly after a jaunt in the car like the one we had just taken. On the afternoon in question she showed no inclination toward sleep, however.

I was proofreading my article. Every minute or so my mother would ask what I was doing. Every minute or so I would tell her that I was finishing up a little work. I would add that if she could nap or read or just be quiet for FIFTEEN MINUTES (I may have raised my voice a tad while saying those words), I would be able to concentrate on her.

She would say, "Of course." And she would mean it. But her sense of time and her short-term memory betrayed her as they always do.

A minute later we would go through the same conversation. Each time I would lose my place in the proofreading.

In desperation, I picked up the phone and called my brother David.

Like most sisters (well, like some sisters—or at any rate like me), I don't say enough nice things about my brother. He is kind, gentle, funny, and knowledgeable. And he has a way with our mother.

He, too, was trying to work, but he made time. Taffy sputtered at him for a little while, telling him I wasn't doing anything with or for her. And then he calmed her down. He is a highly reasonable person. He is also her firstborn (and a boy!) so she is always happy to talk to him.

They chatted for a few minutes about something or other. I wasn't listening; I was too busy reading and typing. When my mother put down the phone, she closed her eyes for ten minutes.

I finished my proofreading, wrote a quick cover note to my editor, and—wonder of wonders—pressed "send" on the computer.

Thank you, David. Thanks to all of you who offer to help. I will be calling on you. And meanwhile, it makes me feel better just to know you're out there!

None of us is alone. And it's not just children whom it takes a village to nurture. Old people and folks in the middle need community, too.

Tuesday, January 25: Fever (but no Peggy Lee)!

Poor Taffy is under the weather.

First, she caught the bug that our whole family has been getting—a nasty cough (I coughed just now as I typed the word "cough") that seems to bring with it a substantial measure of fatigue.

Eventually we realized that she had a urinary-tract infection as well.

Women of her age and condition are prone to the latter—and she is no exception. She gets one every month or two.

Somehow or other I missed this one until it was in full swing. Many times when she gets infections Taffy goes just plain crazy. Unlike some other Alzheimer's sufferers, she doesn't get mean at all—unless she has an infection.

This time around, perhaps because the cough was slowing her down so much, she didn't act crazy. Still, a daughter ought to figure these things out. I did have to change her sheets more than usual—and she wasn't walking as well as she normally does.

For the future I have purchased ... ta da! ... a thermometer so I can check her temperature daily. If she gets a fever, chances are an infection is brewing. And we will head straight to the doctor.

For now, she is on antibiotics. The cough is abating, and the infection had jolly well better be dis-infecting.

At least she and Truffle the dog are getting plenty of rest. And they are both very grateful for the care they receive.

Friday, January 28: Tinky Takes a Bath

Now that Taffy is slowly beginning to feel a little better—thanks to medicine and to the kind wishes friends and blog readers sent for her health and mine—here is an essay that's all about ME!

All the books, web sites, and experts about dementia emphasize the importance of keeping caregivers happy and sane. Actually, I think EVERYONE should be kept happy and sane. We're all caregivers at one time or another.

Our new apartment in Virginia has one of my favorite happiness/sanity enhancers, a convenient bathtub.

In the past couple of homes that my mother and I shared, the bathtubs were adjacent to her room. I was reluctant to take long baths at night for fear of waking her. I was reluctant to take them during the day for fear that she would wander off while I was immersed in the suds.

I didn't go dirty all those months. We did have a shower elsewhere in each house.

To my mind, however, showers are depressingly utilitarian. They get you clean, and that's about all. A bathtub, however, transforms getting clean into a spiritual experience—or at least a luxurious one.

First, I pour in my suds. In my more affluent days I used Vitabath, and I hope to return to its lovely aroma soon. For now cheap bubble bath from a discount store works just fine.

I do a few stretches. I talk to the cat and dog, who are fascinated by the bubbles.

I read. (I've dropped only one book into the water in my life, *The Name of the Rose* in the early 1980s. It ended up a little misshapen but still readable.)

And I contemplate my life and my work.

I used to write in the bathtub. I pictured myself as a plump, female Waldo Lydecker. Lydecker was the memorable acerbic character played by Clifton Webb in the 1944 movie *Laura*.

It was Webb's first big film role, and it came when he was in his mid-50s. Some of us achieve success when we are a little ripe!

Lydecker used his bathroom as an office, mounting his typewriter on a board slung across his marble tub.

I never entertained callers as I wrote in the tub as Lydecker did, but I like to think I had—no, have—a little of his panache.

Unfortunately, now that I write on a laptop computer I am less enthusiastic about writing in the tub. I have a feeling it would be all too easy to ruin the computer or electrocute myself. With my laptop luck, I could probably manage both simultaneously. Machines seem to hate me.

I still brainstorm about my writing as I bathe, however. I come up with a lot of great ideas while soaking. Even when I'm not absolutely brilliant, I enjoy the luxury of the warm, bubbly water. I always arise from the tub refreshed and relaxed.

Of course I'm clean as well. But cleanliness is merely a bonus. We all need to pamper ourselves on a regular basis.

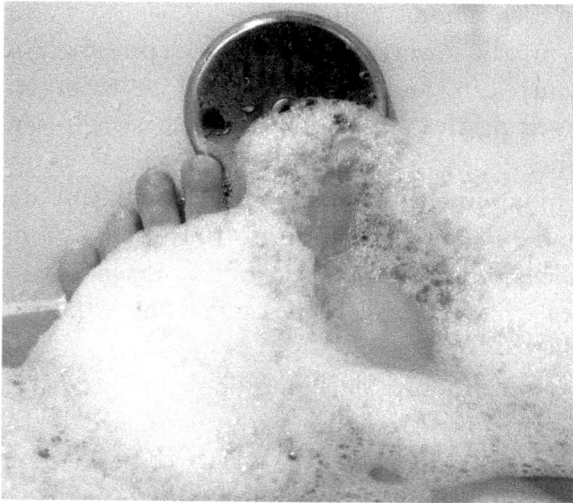

I know the contrast is weak in this picture--but I love thinking about the pink toes in the white tub with the white bubbles!

January Meditation: On Cooking

I mention cooking a fair amount in this book—and I'm tacking a recipe onto the end of each month's chronicles. I thought it might make sense at this point to talk a little about why I love to cook and to discuss the ways in which cooking binds me to Taffy and to other people I love.

First, I cook (and write about food) because it gives me an integrated life. It touches simultaneously on the intellectual, the physical, and the emotional. We think about cooking, food nourishes our bodies, and we have an emotional reaction to food. The phrase "comfort food" has a literal as well as a figurative meaning.

Second, I cook because I was brought up to do so. My family generally prepared meals instead of buying them precooked. When my mother wanted to get to know someone new, or to maintain a friendship she cherished, she shared food. In my childhood home food symbolized family, friendship, and love. It symbolizes them for me today.

That tradition leads me to my paramount reason for cooking. At its best, food doesn't only taste good (a specialty of mine) and look good (not a specialty of mine). It also merges the private (we often cook alone) with the public. I believe that that public component is cooking's essential trait. It connects us to others. It connects us to people with whom and for whom we have cooked. It connects us to people who have shared their recipes and skills with us.

It even connects us to people with whom we have merely sat and chatted while chopping, stirring, or kneading in the kitchen. Thinking back over the years, I remember many conversations that took place during kitchen work, which tends to turn into kin work and friend work.

I remember being instructed by my maternal grandmother on the proper method of washing dishes. She would be appalled at the way I generally wash them today, but she did teach me the correct procedure, and I can use it if I need to!

I remember the care with which she explained in what order—and in what water temperature—glassware, cutlery, plates, and pots should be washed. She was channeling her own adopted mother as she spoke, I am sure.

I remember singing and laughing with my friend Faith as we waited for our penuche to reach the soft-ball stage at my summer home at Singing Brook Farm. It always seemed to take forever. Today when I make fudge by myself it seems to take no time at all. We didn't mind waiting, however. We had stories to tell and songs to sing.

I remember teaching my nephew Michael how to stir a stew when he was so little he had to stand on a stool to reach the stove. As he approaches his teenage years he is less likely to enjoy being in the kitchen so this memory is doubly precious. He was serious … and sweet … and VERY impressed with himself and me!

And I remember arguing and laughing with my mother as we kneaded bread. Or stirred soup. Or chopped vegetables. Or poured booze over fruitcake. Or did any one of a thousand kitchen tasks I have now forgotten. The sense of kinship forged in the kitchen is never forgotten.

My food blog (which I hope will generate another book soon!) is called *In Our Grandmothers' Kitchens*.

Memories like these remind me that one way or another we're almost always in our mothers' and grandmothers' kitchens.

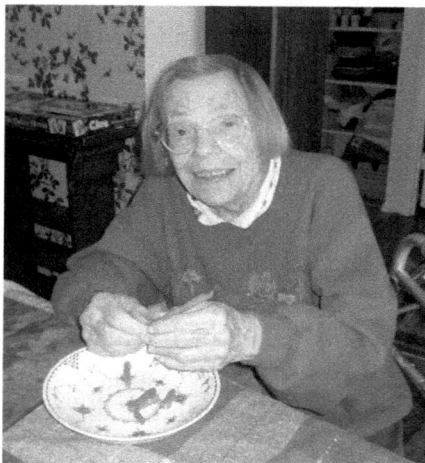

January Recipe: Eleventh Night Vegetable Soup

A note: the proportions of vegetables should depend on how many vegetables you have in the house. And if you don't have these particular vegetables, use what you have.

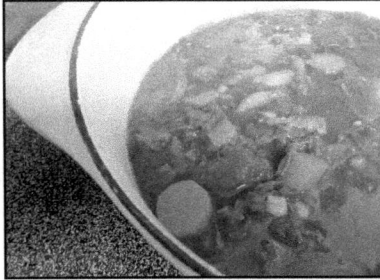

Ingredients:

7 cups sturdy beef stock, preferably homemade
1 handful string beans, trimmed and cut into pieces
3 carrots, trimmed and cut into pieces
1 28-ounce can tomatoes
1-1/2 cups baby potatoes, trimmed and cut into small chunks
1 to 2 cups cooked beef if available (we made the stock from our Christmas roast beef so we had it)
1 to 2 cups corn kernels
salt and pepper to taste
several dollops of red wine
1 handful fresh parsley, finely chopped

Instructions:

Combine the stock, beans, carrots, tomatoes, potatoes, and beef in a large pot. Bring the mixture to a boil; then reduce the heat and simmer, partly covered, for 1/2 hour.

Add the corn and simmer, partly covered, for another 1/2 hour to an hour. If it looks as though you're running low on liquid, cover the soup completely instead of leaving it partly covered.

Taste for seasoning and add salt and pepper as needed. Pour in a little wine and cook, covered, for about 1 hour longer—until the flavors have blended. (Feel free to add a little more wine if you'd like to.) Make sure you don't run out of liquid! Just before serving stir in the parsley. Serves 4 to 6.

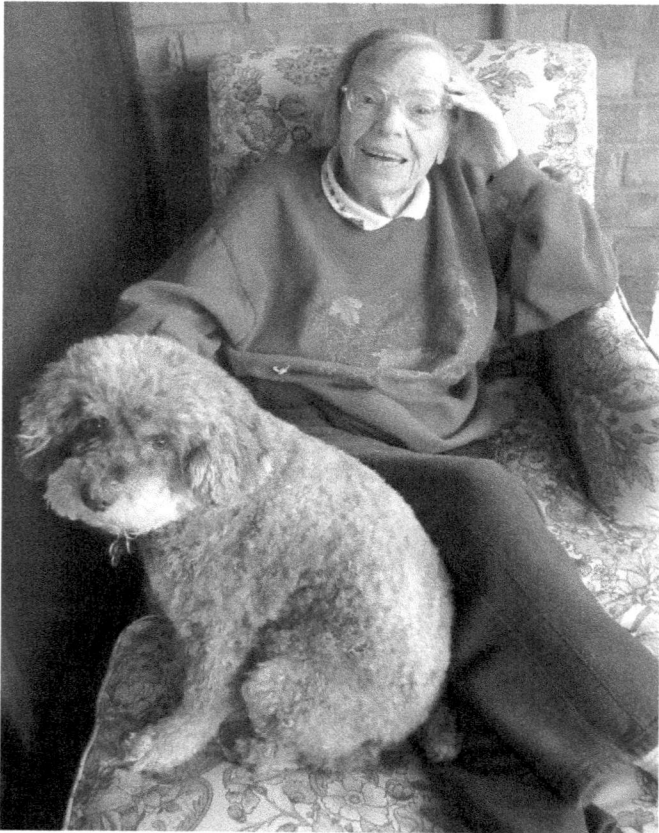

FEBRUARY
Musings

Tuesday, February 1: Time and Memory:
Abe Goes to Jamestown

My mother's current memory problems have prompted me to think about the nature of memory.

I'm not a scientist so I'm not dealing with the ways in which our neurons work to store and retrieve experiences. I'm talking about the way memory feels and works on a daily basis.

I grew up seeing memory operate in contrasting ways. My parents had strikingly different modes of memory and thinking.

Until recently, my mother had an extraordinary long-term memory.

Three years ago she and I drove to Somerville, New Jersey. I was in search of Candyland Crafts, an emporium with what may be the world's largest collection of decorative sprinkles. My mother came along for the ride.

On the way she reminded me that she had worked as a teacher trainee at a school in Somerville for a few months in 1940.

As we left Candyland Crafts with myriad sprinkles she said, "I wonder whether I can find the boarding house I stayed in."

Ten minutes later we were parked in front of it.

I was flabbergasted. I can't find places I visited last month or last year, let alone decades ago.

Before Taffy's dementia took over she and her sister Lura would routinely discuss events of their childhood as though they had taken place just a few days earlier.

(Sometimes, I have to admit, this drove the younger generation crazy because the sisters' memories frequently diverged. It was hard to convince the pair that it really didn't MATTER in 2005 what Aunt Alma had worn to a wedding in 1938.)

Taffy was *The New York Times* of memory, equipped with an archive that went way, way back and was instantly retrievable. In contrast, my father Abe was closer to the CNN of memory. He was strongest on events and people he had encountered within a time frame of a week to a year.

By the time I came along, many of his childhood memories were gone. Only a few vignettes remained from his youth and young adulthood, and those had to be reprocessed frequently; let's call them CNN's most popular historical video clips.

Early in his life he began doing what a lot of older people do—cementing some of his memories by retelling them. Fortunately, he was a wonderful storyteller.

As children, we delighted in hearing about his having been kidnapped on the streets of New York by a man who, true to legend, offered little Abe candy. A family friend spotted the pair about 20 blocks from my father's home and questioned them. The kidnapper ran away, and the child was saved.

My brother and I were also fascinated by the tale of Abe's brainstorm upon receiving a tricycle for his birthday. Why wait for the elevator to descend to the street from his apartment, he reasoned, when his new mode of transportation could get him down the stairs so much more quickly? (Of course, he had scar tissue to reinforce this particular memory.)

Day-to-day events of his younger life were very dim, but these stories lasted into his later years because of their frequent retelling and reshaping.

My own memory is closer to my father's than my mother's. I'm a short- to medium-term girl. It's an asset to me as a journalist; it enables me to focus completely on each story I write. On the other hand, like my father before me I took years and years to complete my Ph.D., in part because it was hard for me to think and plan in the long term.

I'll muse more about memory later. Meanwhile, here's one of my favorites among my father's often told recollections.

Abe, Sergeant York, and Mark Twain

In the 1940s Abe was employed by the Department of Agriculture in Washington. My father was interested in agriculture as a theoretical concept—he went on to get his Ph.D. in agricultural economics—although he had very little practical knowledge of farming.

He sometimes mixed up horses and cows when contemplating them in a pasture, and the lone radish he grew in graduate school was a hard-won achievement.

The department sent him off to do survey research in the South. He ended up one week in Jamestown, Tennessee.

According to my father, the farmers in Jamestown almost immediately took his measure in terms of agricultural knowledge. Shortly after his arrival one of them asked, "Washington, D.C.— what sort of soil do they have up there?"

My father looked clueless and kicked some Jamestown soil with his well shod toe. "Oh, just soil," he replied. "Pretty much like this soil."

The farmers wisely didn't ask him any more questions about agriculture.

Abe eventually found himself asking the farmers a non-agricultural question, however.

Before his arrival he had known Jamestown only as the hometown of Alvin York. York was the famed sharpshooter who received numerous awards (from the Congressional Medal of Honor to the Croix de Guerre) for killing and capturing a ton of Germans during World War I.

When my father arrived in Jamestown, he expected to see many tributes to the military hero, whose story he remembered from the 1941 Gary Cooper film *Sergeant York*.

Instead, over and over he saw the name "Mark Twain." He stayed at the Mark Twain Inn, ate at the Mark Twain Café, and so forth.

Abe was aware that Mark Twain had grown up in Hannibal, Missouri—not in Jamestown, Tennessee. He finally asked residents why Twain's name appeared all over their town. He was informed that Jamestown had been Twain's pre-natal home.

"Alvin York could shoot," said one farmer. "Heck, everybody here can shoot.

"But Mark Twain could write, and that's really something."

Like many of my father's stories, this one may not have been entirely factual. But it certainly rang true.

Friday, February 4: Time and Memory II:
Pros and Cons of My Memory

I noted earlier that I inherited my father's memory, which tended to work best in the short term. This has advantages and disadvantages for me as a caregiver for my mother.

My short-term orientation enables me, like Taffy herself, to take advantage of all the joys life offers us. When she is in a cheerful mood, when we are doing something we love—cooking or singing or reading a poem—we are both absolutely in the moment. And we have a blast.

It means that when she is feeling well and smiling, I smile back without thinking about work I have to do or places I have to go or phone calls I have to make.

On the other hand, my short-term orientation gives changes in my mother's health an ability to surprise me that they wouldn't have if I were better geared toward long-term thinking.

Part of me reads lots of books and talks to lots of people about Alzheimer's and dementia. That part of me SHOULD know what to expect.

But the everyday Tinky is thrown off course every time her mother's health takes a turn for the worse.

It's positive that I don't worry too much about her future. But I ought to be able to plan for it. For the moment, planning is on my to-do list.

Addendum: More about Abe's Trip to Jamestown

After I wrote about my father's habit of cementing some of his longer-term memories by retelling them over and over, my brother reminded me of another, extremely short story my father used to relate about his visit to Jamestown, Tennessee.

(My brother inherited our mother's memory, not our father's, so he tends to recall events and tales of our childhood much better than I do! He may well correct my recollection of Abe's recollection.)

My father's trip to interview farmers in Jamestown lasted through the weekend. On Sundays there was little to do in

Jamestown but go to church. Abe decided to see what churchgoing was like in this rural community.

Sunday worship there turned out to be a serious, soul-searching ritual. Abe was much too polite to say so, but I have a feeling that visiting church was a bit like going to the theater for this Jewish boy from New York.

The preacher was a colorful character known as Brother Timothy. He apparently spent a lot of time exhorting his fellow Jamestowners to join him in resisting Satan.

"And the trouble is, to most of us," intoned Brother Timothy (and here my father's voice would quaver in imitation and he would point with a vigorous finger to an imaginary congregation), "SATAN COMES IN LIQUID FORM!"

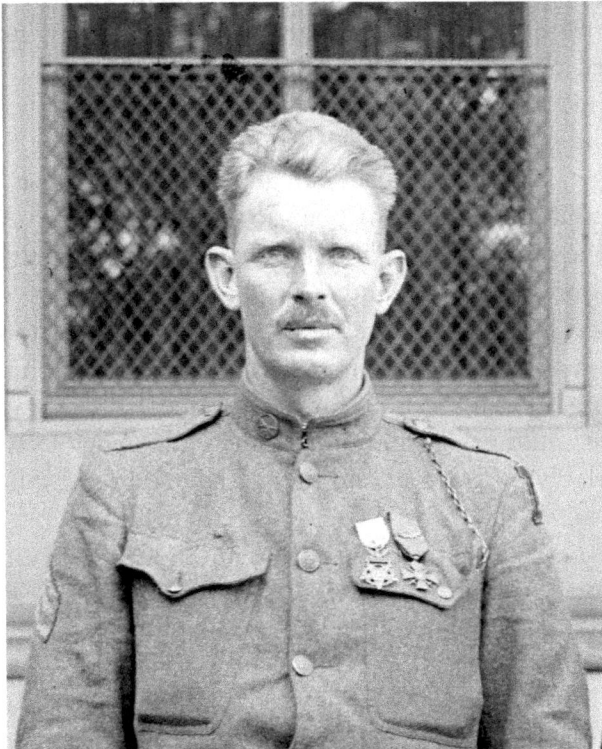

Sergeant York in 1919 (Library of Congress)

Friday, February 11: Puppy Love

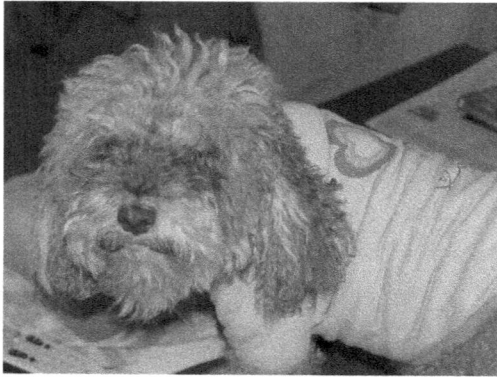

With Valentine's Day looming I thought I'd talk about the importance of love in my mother's life—specifically, puppy love (and kitty love as well). This love is strong and mutual.

I think that if my mother had to move to an assisted-living facility she might not miss me as much as I'd miss her. She would rapidly get used to whatever caregivers she had; she is generally cheerful and grateful for any help from any person.

On the other hand, I think she would be desperately unhappy without our dog, Truffle, and our cat, Lorelei Lee.

Taffy is more likely to recognize them than she is to recognize me. She may not always remember Truffle's name. She has only begun forgetting it recently; for a long time Truffle's was the only name she could call to mind with any consistency. Nevertheless, she invariably looks down and says, "There's my dog. She's a good dog."

Most pet lovers know that caring for and stroking animals can lower blood pressure and stress. Our furry friends also provide undemanding companionship—particularly to individuals who suffer from dementia.

Think about it. To Truffle and Lorelei, my mother's dementia makes little difference to her essence. If they were dependent upon her for meals and exercise, it might matter. I have been their primary caregiver as well as hers for quite a while, however, so they don't expect anything from her but love.

To them, Taffy is actually more appealing now than she was before she got sick. In her prime she was constantly in motion, hardly ever stopping to make a lap yet alone take a nap.

Now she sits or sleeps a lot of the time and always welcomes canine and feline company.

They don't care that she asks the same questions over and over again. They love to be talked to; they have little interest in the substance of her conversation. Let's face it: English is not their first language, although Truffle has quite a large vocabulary.

And, like Taffy, Truffle and Lorelei Lee live in the present. The next caress, the next treat, are all that matters.

She talks to them, sings to them, cuddles them, and rubs them. She also gives them a LOT of food. In exchange, they provide loyalty, companionship, warmth, and unconditional love.

Unlike her human companions, they don't try to make her adhere to any schedules or eat nutritious food or take pills or bathe at certain times or remember a darn thing.

Lorelei and Truffle also make Taffy laugh—which is great medicine for any ailment.

I know that's a cliché, but clichés are often true.

Happy Valentine's Day from all of us........

Tuesday, February 15: Piano Woes

I like to have a piano in the house. I'm a pretty dreadful pianist. Nevertheless, I plonk away on the keys to learn vocal music and accompany myself as I practice singing.

More importantly, to me a piano is like a stove in the kitchen or art on the walls. It is part of what makes a house a home.

When we acquired our apartment in Virginia my sister-in-law Leigh offered us her late mother's 1912 Stieff upright. In its day the Baltimore-based Stieff piano company was known as "the Steinway of the South."

My mother had paid to move this piano to Leigh's home in Virginia in the hope that my nephew Michael might take an interest in learning to play it. (He didn't.)

We cheerfully moved the Stieff into our apartment in Alexandria, where it looked lovely but sounded as though it needed a good tuning.

A musician friend recommended a piano technician named Bruce Anderson. Bruce gave the piano a few weeks to get used to its new environment and then came to tune it.

As he sat on the piano stool he gave us bad news. According to Bruce the poor old Stieff was no longer able to hold a tune. He said he could restring it, put in new pins, and do some bridgework for $4000 to $5000.

Given this cost he suggested we consider buying another piano. He counseled me to look at newer used pianos and get back in touch with him.

I gasped and called my honorary cousin Eric the High-End Piano Guy. Eric concurred with Bruce's assessment. It was time, he said, to bid farewell to the Stieff.

I began visiting showrooms to look at the good used upright pianos available. Sadly for my budget (because I had no budget), these pianos were all in the $5000 range.

Worse than their price was the way they looked. To a piano they were smaller than the Stieff and didn't have its personality. They tended to sport square corners and an unappealing shiny black lacquer finish.

The Stieff is a warm-brown instrument with gentle curves and period trim. It embodies early 20th-century grace and charm. The newer pianos sounded fine, but their outer shells had no charm.

I relayed this information to Cousin Eric, who asked reasonably, "Do you want a musical instrument or a piece of furniture?"

I wanted both.

I began to feel huge amounts of stress.

In fact, while leaving one of the piano showrooms I actually backed the car into a brick wall. Luckily, I was only going one mile per hour so neither the car nor the wall suffered—but the event shook me up.

I don't like to be reminded that my driving is barely better than my piano playing. And hitting a brick wall seemed to be some kind of metaphor.

I called Bruce the Tuner back to ask how long he thought the Stieff would hold up if we paid for the repairs. He said he couldn't make any guarantees and again recommended buying another piano.

I told him that it really pained me to dump a beautiful old piano.

Bruce replied, "Everything has a life, whether it's pianos or people. And it's hard when you get to the end of life. But you have to go on—and be strong."

I thanked him and noticed as I hung up the phone that I was crying.

It was then that I realized that some of my angst about the piano was probably displaced angst about another elderly resident of the apartment.

I don't like to think in the long term, but we are certainly nearing the end of life for Taffy—and getting to the point at which we will just have to go on and be strong.

Amazingly, this story may have a happy ending, or as happy an ending as one gets when dealing with elderly people and elderly pianos.

Bruce the Tuner really is a swell guy. He called back and said he had an idea. If we were willing to put up with having the piano lie around the apartment for a few days on its back, he said, he could apply something called pin glue that might allow the Stieff to be tuned. He wasn't positive it would work, but he was hopeful.

If this technique is successful, the piano still won't last forever—but if I get a humidifier (dry, high-rise apartments are apparently anathema to old pianos) and treat the instrument gently I should be able to keep it going for a while.

Living with an elderly mother and an elderly cat, I would be happy to settle for "a while." It would allow me to dry my tears and enjoy the soulful Stieff—and give me time to think about my piano future.

Friday, February 18: And Now a Few Words from Taffy: "Delhi's Streets"

Here's a contribution from Taffy herself, although it's a few decades old. I love to "hear" her voice in her prime.

I inherited my storytelling talent from my father. I got my writing ability from my mother.

My father sounded great when he talked, but somehow when he wrote things down they could become garbled.

My mother wrote pretty much as she spoke, eloquently and succinctly.

She was also occasionally moved to write a poem. The poem that follows comes from a short collection of her verse titled *My India*.

Taffy adored India—the people, the colors, the air, the food.

My parents lived in India twice.

When my older brother was a baby my father was given a Ford Foundation fellowship to study something or other. (I think his main assignment was to talk to people and report back to the foundation; he was very good at talking to people.)

My parents and brother lived in Mumbai (then known as Bombay). It has always been Taffy's favorite Indian city. She contracted polio during this stay yet she always remembered it with great fondness.

Our family also lived in New Delhi many years later when I was in high school. My mother wrote *My India* during this second sojourn, and it conjures up the India I recall from my youth.

I have a feeling the bustle of Delhi has changed by now. Its streets certainly hold many more cars than they did in the poem.

But I know India is still on the move.

And I like to think of Taffy, saried and combed herself, leaning into the wind as she wrote these words in her beloved India.

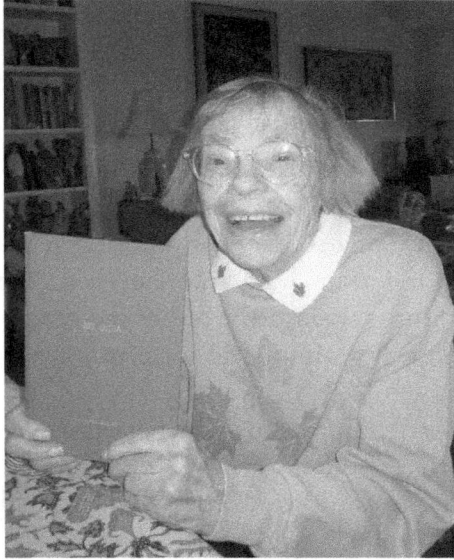

Taffy with her book of poetry

Delhi's Streets

India is on the move.
It is bullock carts and tongas –
Horses and buggies with one seat facing rear.
Bicycles, three abreast on the main streets.
Men, pulling carts of furniture,
And small boys, riding father's bullock cart
At three miles an hour,
Driving home from market
Smiling at sudden manhood.
Taxis and scooter cabs
Zipping along on three wheels,
Open to the breezes.
Buses with people oozing from the doors
And trucks with OK TATA written on the back.
Scooters and bikes whizz by
Each carrying its extra lady passenger
Saried and combed,
Leaning into the wind.

Tuesday, February 22: Imaginary Friends

Generally speaking, my mother is tired at the end of her day and falls asleep quickly.

From time to time, however, I hear her chattering away in her room. Sometimes she mutters for a few minutes. Occasionally she's at it for hours.

My approach to her solitary conversation varies.

About half the time I go into her bedroom to determine whether something is wrong. The rest of the time I leave her alone, hoping that she will go into a deep sleep more quickly if I don't disturb her.

So far I haven't figured out whether either of these strategies works better than the other.

A few nights ago as I heard Taffy talking quietly to herself the phone rang. My brother said he'd love to speak with her if she wasn't asleep.

I explained that she was awake but in chatter mode. I took the phone into her room and put it on "speaker." (She hears better that way.)

David asked her whom she had been talking to. "The children," she explained.

"What children?" David and I wanted to know.

"The children who are here," she replied matter of factly. She went on to describe them. Unfortunately, her description didn't help us figure out what they looked like or where they were in the room.

At first I was taken aback. These apparitions struck me as creepy. I thought of the 2001 film *The Others,* in which young residents of a mysterious house sense the ghostly presence of a child from a different era.

Soon, however, I realized that the situation was closer to that of another film, the whimsical 1950 picture *Harvey.* In this movie James Stewart's character befriends a large white rabbit that is, as my roommate Alice from Dallas used to say, "a Fig Newton of his imagination."

In other words, my mother's "children" were probably imaginary friends.

This makes sense. Taffy has regressed to an age at which imaginary friends are common. We think she perceives herself to be somewhere between two and ten years old, depending on the company and the task at hand.

I didn't have imaginary friends when I was little—unless you count the Academy of Motion Picture Arts and Sciences, whom I thanked frequently for awards in front of my mirror.

I rather envied my friends who enjoyed convenient invisible buddies.

According to Anita Gurian of the NYU Child Study Center, imaginary friends come along "at a time when [children] are beginning to form their own identities and to test the boundaries between fantasy and reality." Gurian posits that the friends help children experiment with different relationships, explore the concept of control, and deal with changes in their lives.

I haven't yet figured out what Taffy's friends do for her. She tends to see them only when she is very sleepy so her descriptions are imprecise.

Perhaps they just keep her company. We don't have a lot of small children around for her to play with.

She certainly has issues with relationships and control, and changes in her life to deal with. And her sense of identity is in flux—as is her perception of the boundary between the real and the not-real.

I'm no longer alarmed when I hear chattering to them. They seem benign. And I'm happy she has someone close to her mental age to talk to.

I am curious, however. If I listen hard enough, perhaps one of these days I'll get a clearer picture.

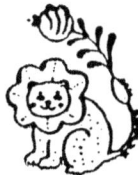

Friday, February 25: LOST!

Almost every family of a person with dementia can tell stories about times at which the patient has wandered off.

In Taffy's case the wandering (often called "eloping" in the medical professions) is most frequent in the summer and fall. The sun calls to her—and off she goes, often surprisingly quickly and quietly for a person using a walker.

Each of our two homes offers advantages and drawbacks when it comes to what I like to call her unauthorized excursions. In Massachusetts we live in a small town so I have help finding her when she toddles off. Neighbors keep their eyes out for her and report in if they spot her making her way up the road, with or without Truffle.

On the other hand, our house there is near lots of uninhabited woods in which she could get REALLY lost. So I still worry. When we return north in the spring I plan to buy some door-knob covers so that she can't open the doors without help. It seems cruel, but the house has four doors, and even though I have put bells on all of them there are times when I don't hear the ringing.

In Virginia we live in an apartment with only one door. The apartment maintenance people have installed a chain high up inside the door (well, high for Taffy or me; we are shrimps) so that she can't take off by herself. I love that chain.

Yet if she DOES somehow get out, getting her home is more difficult than it is in Massachusetts. All the floors in our building look alike. Taffy has no idea what apartment she lives in or even what her married name is. And our building alone houses more people than live in our Massachusetts town so not everyone knows her.

Obviously, I try not to leave her on her own.

Last weekend, however, she was kidnapped. By a mechanical device.

We were (and are) still unpacking and sorting ourselves into the apartment. I had been planning to buy a little recliner so that Taffy could sit in comfort in our tiny sunroom. The sunroom used to be a balcony, but we have enclosed it and crammed it with furniture as is our wont. It's very festive with my Indian canopy on the ceiling—sort of like a colorful overstuffed tent.

I learned that someone on the ninth floor of our building was having a furniture sale on Saturday. Taffy and I went to investigate.

The sale included a two-piece floral chaise longue that had belonged to a 90-year-old woman who was now in smaller quarters and could no longer use it. The chaise was small and comfortable. Taffy tried sitting in it and approved.

The woman holding the sale offered to carry the smaller piece of the chair (the ottoman) to the elevator for us. A neighbor said she would help me carry the chair itself to the elevator and down to our apartment on the sixth floor.

Off we sailed to the elevator. The ottoman was placed in the elevator. Taffy and her walker got in. The neighbor and I picked up the chair.

And then, before we could get it into the elevator, the door just CLOSED. With my poor little mother inside it.

Only one elevator was working that day. I pushed the "down" button and hoped that perhaps it would return with my mother.

When at length it returned neither Taffy nor the ottoman was visible.

The neighbor and I decided that we would take the chair down to our floor; then I would use the stairs to run from floor to floor in search of the missing mother.

Happily, when we arrived at the sixth floor, there was Taffy. Our helpful cleaning woman, Ruth, had happened to be coming into the lobby and had discovered my mother wending her way toward the front door on her way "home."

Ruth told me that someone had put the ottoman in the lobby. She and the neighbor stayed with Taffy while I went to get it.

Obviously, we are going to have to get an I.D. bracelet for my mother in case of future elevator hostilities. And I'm going to have to watch those elevator doors LIKE A HAWK....

February Meditation: Taffy's Youth

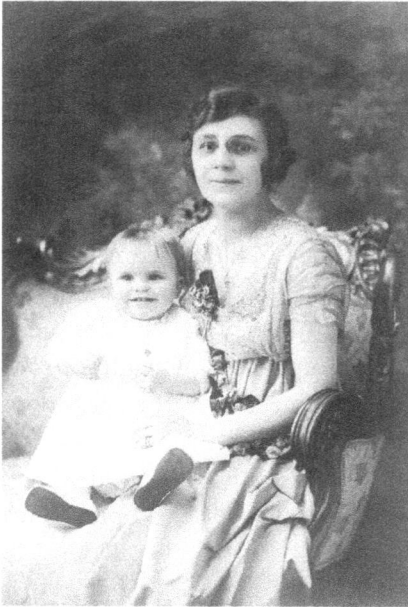

My mother, Janice Hallett Weisblat (a.k.a. Jan or Taffy), was born in 1918 in Brooklyn, New York. Her parents moved to the suburb of Maplewood, New Jersey, when she was about two, and she maintained a residence in New Jersey for most of her life.

Bruce and Clara Hallett adored baby Janice. As their first child she received all the attention first children customarily expect. Her baby book begins:

"This is a record of the child-life of Janice Elizabeth Hallett, our darling baby who keeps her mother everlastingly going. She first smiled October 31st at the age of five weeks and giggled aloud February 4th."

Bruce was a lawyer; Clara was a homemaker and amateur singer. (Her husband called her "the little girl with the big voice.") Janice's mother was quiet but loving and encouraged her daughter to invite friends to the house; an orphan, Clara had never enjoyed this luxury as a little girl. Bruce was an affectionate father but a strict one.

"He was a disciplinarian—expected immediate obedience!" my mother wrote late in life. "I can remember being put in the corner and saying to myself, 'I'll never speak to my daddy again.' Ten minutes later I was on his lap and hugging him."

Little Janice was something of a prodigy and was routinely asked by her parents to recite poetry to guests from the age of two on. She grew up knowing she was smart and knowing she was loved.

Her childhood was secure with few pressures and many novelties as she observed the world change around her. She listened to Lindbergh's historic landing in Paris in 1927 on a radio with earphones, learned to use a rudimentary telephone, went to the movies to see exciting serials on Saturdays, and waved at pilots in monoplanes so close you could see their faces in the sky.

She played tag and hide-and-seek. She swam and gazed at cloud formations in the skies. She put on plays for the neighborhood. The Halletts gathered around the piano on Saturday evenings for sing-alongs and enjoyed Sunday rides in their car.

Taffy was friendly and enthusiastic as a child, with a flair for the dramatic. She briefly studied the violin and enjoyed wandering around the town playing melancholy tunes on the instrument, imagining the reactions of passersby to this touching sight. When she saw an African American on the street, she soulfully asked, "Don't you just LOVE Abraham Lincoln?"

Luckily, the adults around her did little to quash her … with one exception. Her family made a yearly pilgrimage in the summer to the home of Calvin Coolidge in Plymouth, Vermont. To their surprise on one visit the president was in residence.

Little Janice spotted him on the side of the road and ran up to accost him. (This was obviously before the Secret Service started protecting our chief executives around the clock.) "Hello, Mr. President! Hello, Mr. President!" she cried with her widest smile.

Coolidge looked down grimly for a moment and then dismissed her with a curt "Good day, little girl." He turned on his heel and headed back into his house.

As time went by the family expanded. When Janice was two her brother Bruce came along—her forever playmate, beloved by his mother because he was a boy and by his father because he was an athlete.

When she was nine her sister Lura was born. Although Janice occasionally resented having to take care of her little sister, like her parents and brother she loved the beautiful, curly-haired baby of the family.

Two groups of older relatives and their houses figured prominently in young Janice's sense of home and family. First, her mother's two sisters, Alma and Charlotte, played a crucial part in the Hallett clan. Clara, Alma, and Charlotte had been orphaned when they were very young, and as the eldest Alma worked hard to keep the sisters in touch through the years.

When Bruce Hallett married Clara, he was made to understand that he was in a sense marrying all three sisters. Holidays were divided up among the siblings: Clara hosted Christmas, Charlotte did Thanksgiving, and Alma rang in the new year. Summers were also special times in which the sisters and their families bonded.

A large cushiony sort of person, Alma offered hugs and comfort whenever they were needed. The baby of the family, Charlotte was a spunky fighter all her life. She identified with lively little Janice and often joked that Jan was her true daughter while her own staid Young Charlotte should have been born to the prim Clara.

In her 80s Aunt Charlotte discovered some young neighborhood toughs in Jersey City picking on a smaller boy. "Put up your dukes!" she told the hooligans, assuming a boxing stance. They were more surprised than frightened, but they withdrew. Charlotte passed her "put up your dukes" attitude on to her niece.

My mother's other close relatives were her mother's adoptive parents, Lura and George Thrall. Her heart's home was the Thralls' house on North Main Street in Rutland, Vermont. The whole family called them Aunt Lura and Uncle George. Taffy adored them.

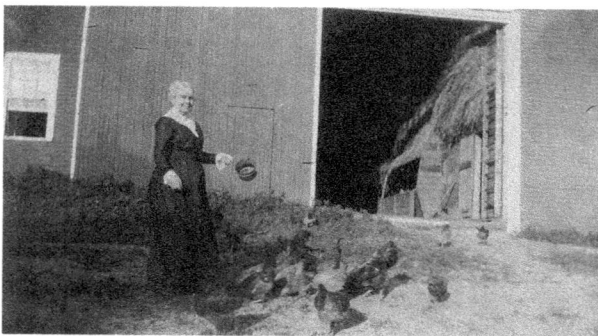

*Aunt Lura
feeds her
chickens.*

After July 4 every year my grandmother and her children went north to spend the rest of summer's sunny days in the Thralls' sprawling farmhouse. (My grandfather stayed in New Jersey to continue working, although he rode the train up for visits.)

In her 50s Taffy wrote a brief family history. In it she recalled idyllic days in Rutland.

At noon, for I am four or five and it is 1923, Aunt Lura or Mother will go to the door and ring the big farm bell which later came down to Maplewood and was used to call us children in from play. Uncle George and the hired man will come in from the field, and Gladys [the hired girl], Mother and Aunt Lura will have the table all set in the big dining room and the food piping hot. Our vegetables come from the garden up in the field where Alex, the hired man, has cleared a 50 by 100 foot plot, and we have made our chicken and our cottage cheese. We may also have biscuits and home made bread and butter pickles.

The big old grandfather clock ticks away in the corner. Uncle George bows his head. "For what we are to receive, Oh Lord, make us truly grateful." Everyone is hungry. Bruce is little so he sits near mother but I am a big girl so I will sit near Gladys. For dessert we have raspberry pie which we all love. I eat my piece and get out all the raspberries but the crust is delicious too.

Uncle George winks at me and says, "Pick it up in your fingers. That's the very best way." But as he starts to demonstrate and I copy him, Aunt Lura is horrified. "Now, George, don't you teach that child bad manners."

For the [last three months of first grade] I went down the hill to Lincoln School in Rutland, a school Mother had attended. I was a real little smart aleck. I was bright in school, I knew how to read, and I was well ahead of the other children in my class. I was also only there for a short time. As a result, I took all kinds of liberties.

I wandered from class to class, dropping in on the fourth grade to see my friend, Elizabeth Sherman, if I felt so inclined, and bragged about how I answered an arithmetic problem when a fourth grade boy did not know the answer. I recited "The owl and the pussycat went to sea......" to anyone who would listen; in short, I was quite a showoff.

Except for this brief foray into education in Vermont, Taffy went to public school in New Jersey. She went on to attend Mount Holyoke College in South Hadley, Massachusetts. I'll discuss that more later.

When Taffy turned 21 a few months after graduation from college her parents wrote her long letters promising that her birthday present, her own radio, would be delivered soon. Her mother shared neighborhood and household news—a friend's job uncertainty, young Lura's sickness, a dress that had to be returned to the store. Her father, who loved to mark any occasion with deep thoughts, shared life advice with his "Punkins."

"Sir Isaac Newton was a dreamer," wrote my grandfather. "If he hadn't been, the falling apple wouldn't have inspired him to *think*. The trick is to dream and be practical too. The great lawyers, doctors, musicians, teachers, philosophers, for the most part have been great because of their ability to translate their dreams to practical application."

His daughter was to take this advice to heart throughout her life, combining a romantic spirit with ruthless common sense.

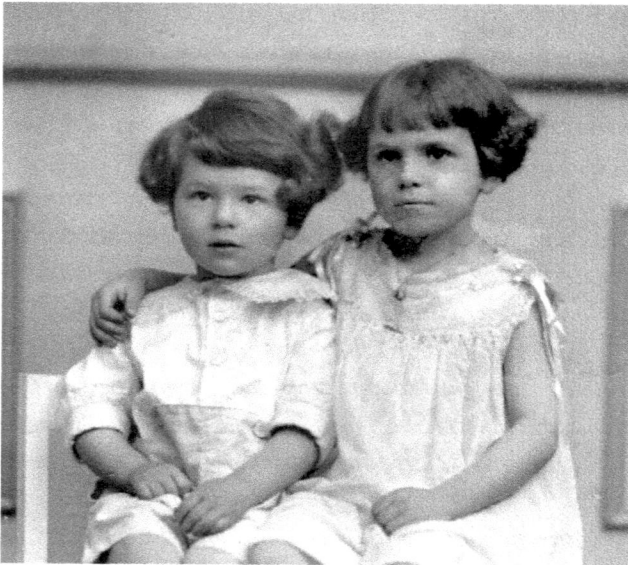

Little Janice (right) with brother Bruce

February Recipe: Ghost Farm Cookies

As a child and in her old age, Taffy was a fiend for cookies—the simpler the better.

Cookie recipes don't get much simpler than this one from Jody Cothey, a resident of our town in Massachusetts who wears A LOT of hats. She and her husband Edward run Tregellys Fiber Farm. There they raise yaks, Icelandic sheep, Bactrian camels, and several dogs as well as other exotic and non-exotic animals.

Under the name Pamela Stewart, Jody also writes poetry. Her most recent book of poems is called *Ghost Farm*.

Ingredients:

1 cup (2 sticks) sweet butter at room temperature
1/2 cup dark (or light!) brown sugar, firmly packed
1/4 teaspoon baking soda
2 cups flour

Instructions:

Preheat the oven to 325 degrees. Cream together the butter, brown sugar, and soda. Stir in 1 cup of the flour. Transfer the dough to a board (on which you have sprinkled part of the second cup of flour!) and knead it.

Knead in the remaining flour. The dough will be quite stiff by the time you finish incorporating all the flour.

Jody suggests a number of ways in which to shape her cookies, including rolling them out and cutting them. Here's what I do: I roll my dough into three logs and cut each log into thin cylinders. I then press the cylinders into little flat circles.

Place the cookies on an ungreased cookie sheet and bake them for 15 to 20 minutes. Let them cool on the cookie sheet for a few minutes before transferring them to a wire rack to finish cooling.

Makes about 24 cookies (more or less, depending on how big you cut/roll them).

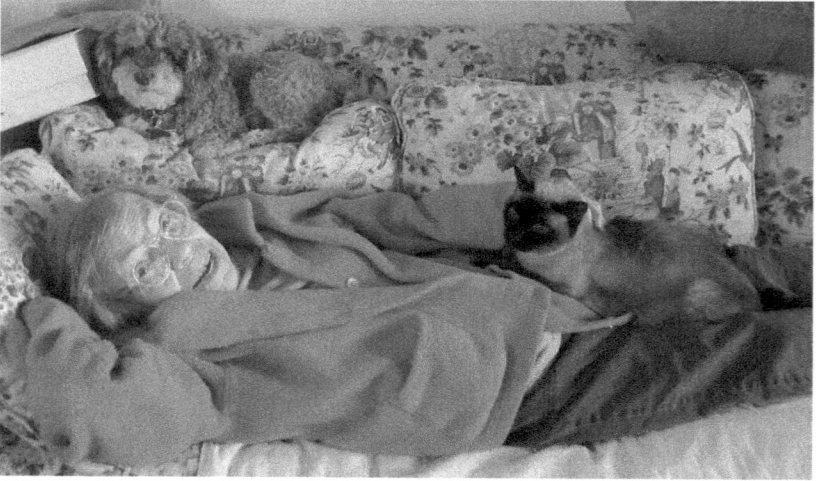

Lots of naps were taken during the month of March.

MARCH
A Rough Spring

Thursday, March 10: Holding On/Holding Out in Church

Since our move to Virginia my mother and I have made noises from time to time about going to church.

So far I have auditioned four churches in Alexandria. The experience has left me with a feeling that we're not destined to attend a church here very much. By the time we combine what I'm looking for in a church with what my mother needs in one, the task of finding a place to worship becomes daunting.

Nevertheless, the exercise of looking at churches and reacting to them has taught me a lot about those wants and needs.

My mother's requirements begin with the physical. She needs a church with convenient parking and easy access for a not-too-strong person who uses a walker.

She also appreciates a minister and congregation who are welcoming and who understand someone who tends to ask questions in the middle of the service such as "Is she [meaning the minister] someone's mommy?"

The sound system must amplify voices sufficiently for a slightly deaf person. This requirement is actually becoming less important these days since all the amplification in the world can't make Taffy's brain process what she hears, but she still likes to be able to hear.

Finally, she needs familiarity—the Lord's Prayer, hymns she has sung all her life, and a sense of belonging.

Some of my own requirements in a church might have been expected. I'm looking for a good choir (we chanteuses worship to a great extent with our voices), a sense of community (churches are all about people), and a minister whose heart is in the right place. It's helpful if he or she is also smart and has a sense of humor.

A couple of the things I seem to be looking for have taken me by surprise. Unexpectedly for a person who is verbal rather than visual, I realized after visiting a couple of soulless modern structures that I value architecture in a church.

One spends a lot of time in church quietly meditating so one's surroundings are important. And it's easier to feel close to the divine in a building that at least tries to approach divinity in its design.

Even more surprisingly, since I was brought up Unitarian, I seem to like a little theology and ritual. (I guess I've been attending Christian churches too long!)

As you can see, if you put those two sets of requirements together, you have A LOT of requirements.

My church of choice if I were on my own would be the Old Presbyterian Meeting House in Old Town Alexandria, Virginia, which I visited one Sunday a while back when my brother was available to keep our mother company.

This church's talented choir sings challenging music. Its liturgy is familiar. Its people seem friendly. Its minister is thoughtful and quirky. (During his sermon he managed to touch on topics from country music to the Harlem Renaissance, quoting both Willie Nelson and Langston Hughes.) And its architecture—late 18th century—is ideal, gracious but not overwhelming.

Unfortunately, parking downtown is limited so there is really no way to get Taffy into this church.

I was hoping that the local Unitarian church might offer a compromise I could live with. The staff and congregation couldn't be friendlier. And although the building is new its design is attractive, particularly to one who tries VERY hard to forget that she has seen the Old Meetinghouse.

The choir is robust. And handicapped parking abounds.

Unfortunately, when we went there on Sunday the church did not "take."

It had moveable chairs rather than pews so it was hard for Taffy to stand up to sing hymns; she had no sturdy wooden railing to lean on. I told her she didn't need to stand up, but if everyone else stands she wants to.

The choir sounded a bit muddy, perhaps in part because of the room's acoustics (another reason why architecture is important!).

Taffy was taken aback by the fact that the hymns were unfamiliar. When I was a child in a Unitarian church, we sang standard Protestant hymns with the words changed to de-emphasize Christ and the Trinity.

The church we attended on Sunday had a new hymnal with peppy but rather simplistic (mostly) new songs that didn't mention God at all. Taffy was stymied.

As for me, I was stymied by the theology or lack thereof. Appealingly, the minister supported humanity and social justice, but not mentioning God at all in a church seemed a bit extreme to me.

She ended her prayers (or meditations or whatever you want to call them) with the expression "Blessed Be."

This brought out the pedant in me. When I taught writing I was very aggressive when it came to stamping out the passive voice. I can stand it on occasion—and I was certainly intrigued when a Chinese colleague told me that he thought the American critique of the passive voice was linguistic cultural imperialism—but I wanted my students to understand that their word choices had consequences.

The passive voice is sloppy and wordy. It also often wipes out agency. Saying, for example, that civilians have been killed in a conflict avoids naming the killers.

To me the phrase "Blessed Be" implies that someone or something is doing the blessing. Not specifying who or what annoys me, to put it mildly.

Somewhere in the middle of the service on Sunday Taffy reached out and grabbed my left hand very tightly with both of her hands. She didn't let go until after the benediction. Clearly, the service spoke to neither of us.

So for the moment we'll spend Sunday mornings reading and chatting. And we'll bide our time until we get back to our lovely 19th-century Congregational church in Massachusetts.

Taffy doesn't understand a word Cara, our minister, utters from the pulpit there. But she can hum the hymns. And whenever she goes to church she is greeted with love by Cara and the congregation. She leaves Sunday-morning services with a smile on her face.

I sing in the choir, listen with interest to Cara, and feel free to avoid taking communion. I'll probably never be Christian enough to embrace the bread and the cup. But I feel comfortable listening to the organ and gazing at the Tiffany windows while others sip and nibble.

That's not a church compromise. That's a church home.

Friday, March 18: We Are Siamese, If You Please

Our family's feline elderly lady injured herself a few days ago. Poor Siamese Lorelei Lee has been limping around the apartment. Her left rear leg is in the air whenever possible, and her face reveals the sorrow and resignation of an Oriental martyr.

I should admit that it's possible that I am responsible for this injury. Princess Lorelei started throwing up at four in the morning on a night during which Queen Taffy wasn't sleeping very well. (Lorelei has had a tendency to throw up all her life.)

I tossed her (Lorelei, not Taffy) off the bed to avoid having to change the bedding in the middle of the night. I assumed she landed on her feet since she IS a cat—but it's possible that she didn't. She is indeed a cat, but she's also almost 20.

In the morning I noticed the limp and the look. I felt like a terrible cat caregiver. I have now placed a towel on the bed so that I can pop the cat onto it *very gently* when I hear retching in the night.

In a flurry of concern and guilt I took Lorelei Lee to the doctor the next day while my brother kept an eye on Taffy.

Luckily, nothing is broken, but parts of the poor kitty are definitely sore.

In fact, the vet couldn't entirely limit the pain to LL's leg since her highness gave the poor woman grouchy looks when she touched the delicate feline back as well as the sore feline ankle.

"It's really hard to distinguish pain from annoyance in a 19-year-old Siamese cat," said Dr. MacDonald. We sang a chorus of "The Siamese Cat Song" from *Lady and the Tramp*.

As I drove home with a cranky cat and a bottle of anti-inflammatory pills I pondered the parallels between my two old ladies.

My mother seldom expresses pain outright. Like Lorelei Lee, she does get downright grumpy when something is wrong, however. In fact, it's just about the only sign that anything IS wrong.

Taffy has been agitated of late. She is asking for her mother even more than usual, and on many days and nights she has a lot of trouble sleeping.

I had thought that this was just a sign of a new stage or mini-stage in her dementia. Perhaps, however, it indicates that she is hurting somewhere, somehow.

Luckily, she is scheduled to go to two doctors next week. I hope together we can figure out what if anything is wrong with her.

I doubt that either her urologist or her regular doctor will sing, "We are Siamese, if you please."

Nevertheless, I'd love to hear them try.

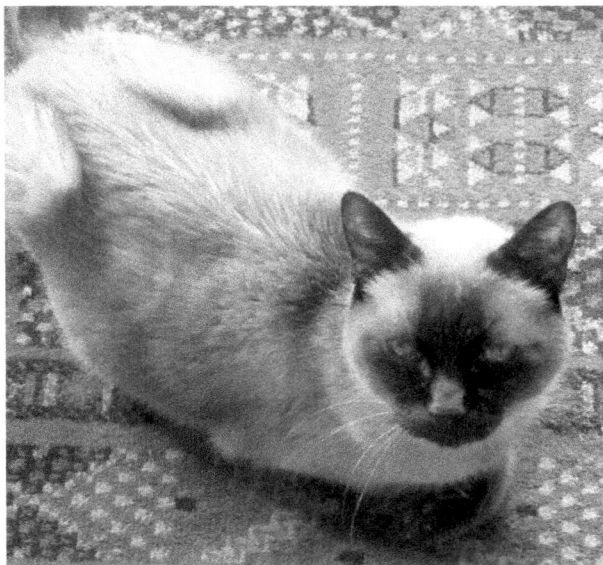

Thursday, March 24: Singing Along

My mother has always loved music and singing.

Over the years she wasn't much of a complainer. I never heard her talk negatively about her experience with polio in her mid 30s. (She caught the disease shortly before the vaccine was introduced.)

Pretty much the only thing I ever heard her grumble about, in fact, was losing her voice.

It happened about 50 years ago. She had a bad cold but sang with gusto at a party one night.

The next morning her speaking voice was lower. And her singing voice had been reduced to a four-note range.

Years later she was told that she had developed polyps on her throat. She had them removed surgically at that point, but the operation failed to restore her voice.

Taffy was less devastated than Julie Andrews was in a similar situation. Unlike Andrews, she had never had a four-octave range. Nevertheless, singing had been a major part of her life. Although she continued to sing in a very pleasant if limited way she always longed wistfully for the voice of her youth.

Today music is still something she can enjoy.

In the past few weeks I have made more of an effort than usual to practice my singing since our local music group sponsored a Saint Patrick's Day sing-along last Thursday at our apartment complex's community center. Naturally, I was assigned a solo.

And naturally, I wanted to perform as well as I could.

I'm not brilliant when it comes to vocal exercises. I do know, however, that the best way to sing well at an event is to have sung every day for at least two weeks beforehand.

So every afternoon in the days before the concert, after Taffy's nap (if she took one, and naturally I loved it if she did!), I practiced several songs as well as my assigned solo, "An Irish Lullaby."

It worked so well that we have continued the rehearsals after the concert—at which Taffy sang along enthusiastically.

In general, my repertoire coincides with the music my mother sang as a young woman. I don't sing a lot of numbers that were written after 1960. So much of what I sing is familiar to her.

Taffy waves her hands to the music, hums or sings along as well as she can, and occasionally dances.

She even seems to learn the music and lyrics of unfamiliar songs, although she has trouble absorbing new material presented in any other format. This behavior accords with a recent study conducted at Boston University in which patients with dementia retained information better when it was set to music.

There's something magical about music for both of us. It taps into a part of Taffy's memory and spirit that doesn't come out all the time.

And it makes me feel pretty darn wonderful as well.

(Did I mention that my solo was fabulous? My neighbors clustered around me, and one said, "I didn't realize we had an amazing coloratura soprano in the building." I'm not quite a coloratura, but who am I to contradict a neighbor? I certainly couldn't argue with the "amazing" part of her description.)

Even the pets enjoy listening.

They're enjoying eating leftover Saint Patrick's Day soda bread with Taffy as well.

Too-ra-loo-ra-loo-ral. That's an Irish lullaby.

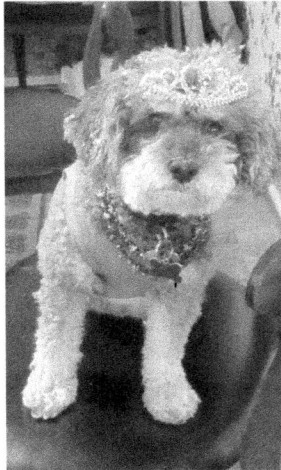

Truffle dressed up for Saint Patrick's Day.
Her shirt says, "Pet me. I'm Irish."

Tuesday, March 29: Smiles on Our Faces

Things have been a bit rocky of late at the Casa Weisblat.

At first I thought my mother was on an upswing. She began to act decidedly perky. She went for lots of walks, did her exercises, and even tried to leave her walker behind on occasion.

Soon, however, I realized that the perkiness had a downside. It was not ordinary perkiness but rather perkiness born of anxiety.

Taffy started having trouble taking naps.

Then she started having trouble sleeping at night.

I have noted before that her occasional sleeplessness is the hardest thing for me to handle. I know there are people who can get by with very little sleep. I don't happen to be one of them.

The worst night was one during which she was convinced that someone was lurking either in or just outside the apartment intending to kill us. She became desperate when I wanted to take the dog out for a walk.

Unfortunately, the dog was suffering from a stomach bug and had major diarrhea. It would be hard to say who had the worst time that night—Taffy, Truffle, or Tinky. (I vote for Tinky, but I'm sure each of the others could make a good case for herself.)

As I noted in my recent entry about the ailments of our elderly cat, Lorelei Lee, Taffy had doctors' appointments last week.

When we arrived at the doctor's office we discovered that—sure enough—Taffy had another urinary-tract infection.

The doctors are still trying to figure out how she contracted the darn thing while taking preventive antibiotics, but meanwhile the medicine they gave her for the infection is working its magic.

She is sleeping a lot more. The circles underneath everyone's eyes are beginning to disappear. (It helps that Lorelei and Truffle are on the mend as well.)

A couple of nights ago Taffy called me into her room.

"I just wanted to say that I'm glad I'm your niece," she told me. (Well, at least she remembers that we're related.) "I can watch you and learn how to do things from you."

"We can learn from each other," I told her with a hug.

A huge grin appeared on her face, she told me she loved me, and she popped back into bed. It was one of those moments that make the harder times worthwhile.

I even smiled at her when she woke up the next morning before seven. I sent her back to bed to try to sleep a little more ... but I smiled.

We are definitely learning from each other. Mother and daughter or niece and aunt: the definition of our relationship shifts by the day. Its essence remains the same. We talk. We receive diagnoses that are both full and bereft of meaning. We smile at each other.

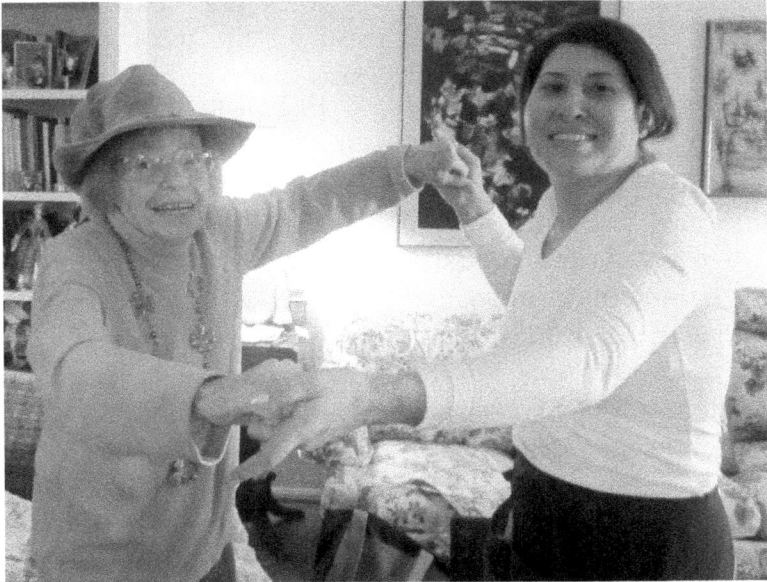

An impromptu dance with Ruth the cleaning woman

March Meditation: Taffy and the Garden State

Often as I listened to my mother long for her childhood home in Maplewood, New Jersey, I was reminded of the strong attachment she felt to the state of New Jersey overall.

In general, Taffy had an inexhaustible sense of humor. That humor took a breather, however, when she heard derogatory jokes about New Jersey. She was dismayed that anyone could think poorly of her home state. "The people who disparage New Jersey," she would say, "have only seen the state from the New Jersey Turnpike. If they got off the highway and looked around, they would appreciate it as I do."

She was particularly indignant when she viewed the Pace Picante Sauce television commercials of the 1980s and 1990s. The ads' cowboy heroes derided salsa made in her home state, pronouncing the words "New Jersey!" with biting southwestern scorn. I tried in vain to explain that the point was not that cowboys disliked New Jersey but that salsa from that state wasn't necessarily authentic.

In a way, she was right. The Pace commercials worked in large part because American popular culture has a stereotypical view of New Jersey that is unflattering. The state is known for its industry and its crowds. Residents are portrayed as loud and rude. The women invariably have big hair and wear too much makeup. And many of the men seem to be involved in organized crime.

Hair and makeup could hardly be more minimal than Taffy's, and New Jersey's face in popular culture is not, in general, that of the state she knew growing up. She didn't come across a lot of Mafiosi or industrial pollution or people with accents like Danny DeVito's. Her own accent was what teachers in drama schools term "Eastern Seaboard" (or at least it's what they termed it when I took acting classes several decades ago!), a way of speaking that is relatively free of regional dialect. Her voice made her sound like a cross between Orson Welles and Judy Garland.

And she came from a culture of civility. The Maplewood in which Taffy grew up was a typical mid-sized American village of the period. She moved to the town during its largest decade of growth. Her parents were the first owners of the house to which they moved from Brooklyn when she was a toddler.

Young Janice could walk or ride her bicycle downtown, where she was familiar with the proprietors of the grocery store, the bakery, the dry cleaner, the stationer, and the hardware store. Her bank account number was under 1000. (She was devastated when the bank was purchased by a larger bank in the 1980s and she was given a large, impersonal account number.)

Her father was active in civic affairs, advising Maplewood's mayor on policy matters. Her mother was a pillar of the local Methodist church and the woman's club. Both her parents were mainstays of the Maplewood Country Club. They believed that a community thrives when its residents participate in it.

All the local kids slid down the same big hill on snow days. And every family in town attended the town's annual Independence Day celebration. Later in life Taffy recalled "races in the morning, the circus in the afternoon, and singing and fireworks at nine." She added, "We went home later and caught fireflies, which we put in glass jars till morning."

Taffy knew that Northern New Jersey was becoming increasingly urban. She visited her aunt in Jersey City frequently, and she shopped for clothing in Newark. Nevertheless, the New Jersey she knew still had plenty of farms (the section of Maplewood known as Hilton was famed for its Hiltonberries, particularly succulent strawberries). And it offered an idyllic small-town atmosphere to growing families.

One could argue that the Maplewood of Taffy's childhood and youth was elitist. Nevertheless, she came out of it with a strong commitment to diversity and civil rights. So the town's fathers and mothers must have been doing something right.

To the end Taffy defended her home state as friendly, even cozy, whenever she could. She encouraged me to be proud of having been born there. And she showed no patience at all with New Jersey's detractors.

I am still tickled when I see the old Pace commercials on YouTube. I freely admit that I was born in New Jersey, however. And I have a fondness for the state, a fondness nurtured by one of its most loyal daughters.

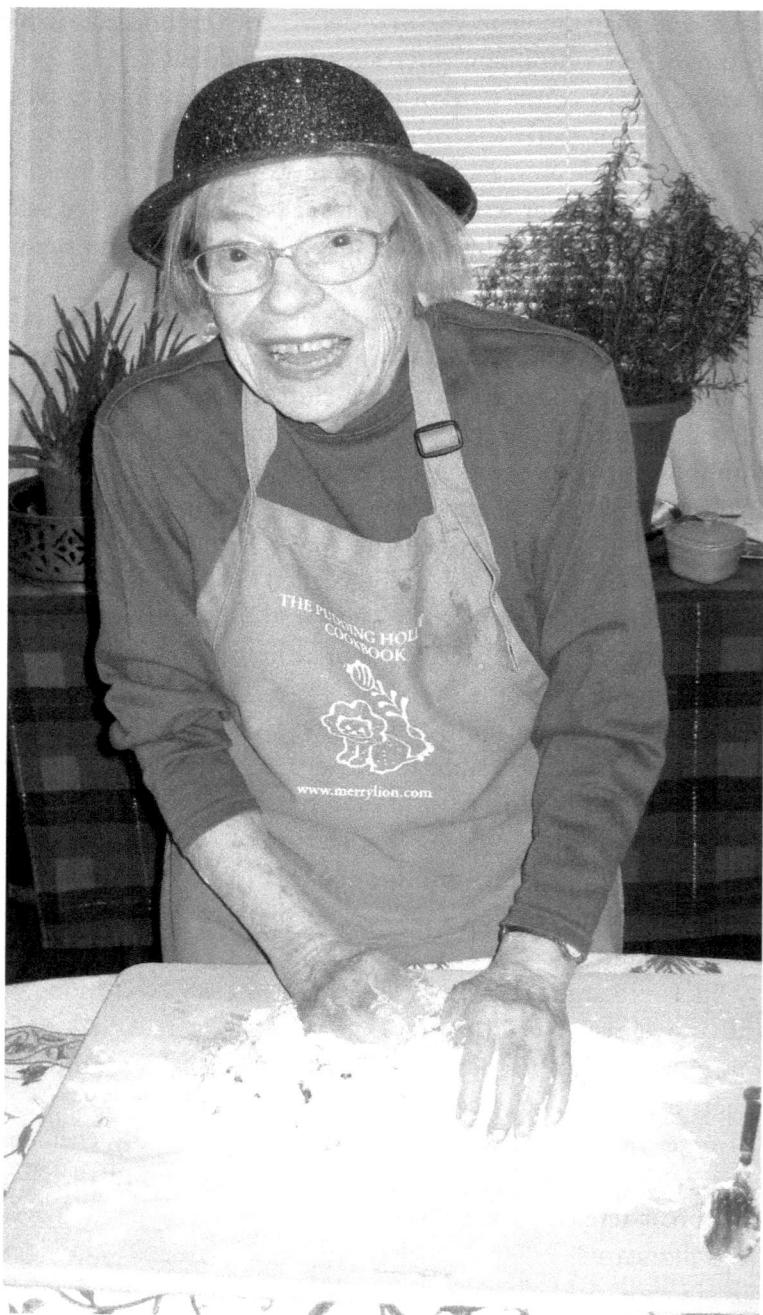

Taffy kneading soda bread in 2009

March Recipe: Irish Cottage Soda Bread

This March-appropriate recipe comes from a now defunct Irish shop in Summit, New Jersey, in which Taffy loved to browse. "My Irish Cottage" used to hold a yearly contest to see which customer could produce the tastiest soda bread. A version of this recipe took first place several years back, and Taffy and I made it every Saint Patrick's Day thereafter. She was our household's designated kneader.

Ingredients:

4 cups flour
1/4 cup sugar
1 teaspoon salt
1 teaspoon baking powder
1/4 cup (1/2 stick) cold butter, cut into six pieces
1 cup dried cranberries (you may substitute raisins if you like)
1 egg
1-1/3 cups buttermilk
1 teaspoon baking soda
green sprinkles (optional)

Instructions:

Preheat the oven to 375 degrees. Grease a large cookie sheet or line it with parchment paper or a silicone mat.

In a bowl, combine the flour, sugar, salt, and baking powder. With two knives or a pastry blender cut in the butter. When you are finished there should be only tiny bits of butter left. Stir in the cranberries.

In a separate bowl whisk together the egg, buttermilk, and baking soda. Combine them with the other mixture—don't mix the dough too much—and form the combination into a ball.

On a wooden board that is lightly floured, knead the dough for three to five minutes. Form the bread into two round mounds, place them on the greased cookie sheet, and make a cross with a serrated knife in the center of each. Throw on sprinkles if you like. Bake the mounds until they are golden brown in spots, about 35 to 40 minutes.

Makes 2 loaves.

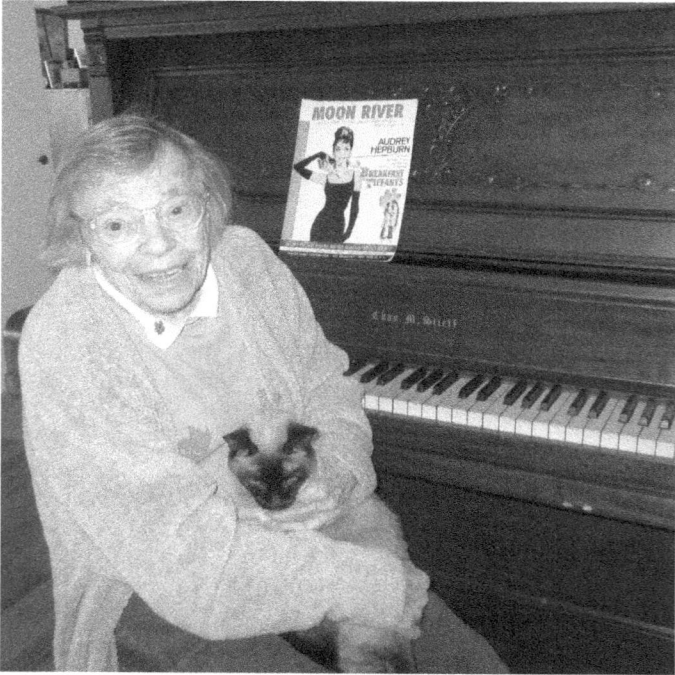

APRIL
Ups and Downs

Friday, April 1: The Best Medicine

When I was a child my family loved to spend time with our cousins in the Netherlands, the Brauns.

The Brauns were a fun clan—they always sent my brother and me chocolate at Christmas!—made even more special by the fact that they represented my father's only remaining family in Europe.

(My father came to this country in 1920 when he was almost two years old. Most of his relatives either immigrated to the U.S. or died in the Holocaust. The Brauns were hidden by Catholics throughout the Nazi occupation of Holland, and I believe they eventually converted from Judaism to Christianity.)

During one memorable visit the Brauns took us to see a fascinating Dutch social experiment—a planned community that featured rows of apartments. The buildings were two stories high.

Elders lived in the lower stories. Families with children lived in the upper stories. The rationale was that both older people and very young people benefit from being in frequent contact with each other.

I don't know whether this community still exists. I hope it does.

I was reminded of it this week when I saw an example of the magic of intergenerational contact.

My mother is still recovering from her most recent infection, and she tends to be sleepy and a little confused. On Tuesday, however, she got back some of her customary focus when our friend Joan Miller Sutton came to visit.

Joan works with seniors and has a definite way with them. In the year or so that we have known her she has recommended doctors, therapists, and aides for Taffy. Joan is clearly interested in older people, and they respond to her vivacity with enthusiasm. She tends to get more memories and more smiles out of my mother than just about anyone else we know.

This week Joan outdid herself in terms of stimulation by bringing along her two-month-old baby, Wyatt.

My mother couldn't take her eyes off the baby. She told him how good he was, examined his perfect little toes, held him, and generally had a wonderful time.

Even Truffle found the baby fascinating. As for me, I'm a sucker for anything small and cute—and they don't come much smaller or cuter than Wyatt.

Our friend Susan has promised to bring her baby Joshua to visit when we get back to Massachusetts so my mother can have another dose of baby magic.

If we could just bottle the feeling she gets when she's with the very young, it would be a lot more effective for curing what ails her than most of the pills she takes.

Wednesday, April 6: Prognosis Positive!

Several weeks back I shared bad news about the piano Taffy and I had been given by my sister-in-law Leigh.

We discovered that our Stieff upright, built in 1912, had several structural difficulties. The worst problem was that the pins used to tune the strings no longer fit into their holes (or whatever the things are called in piano-technician terminology).

So the piano was untunable.

I deal with human and feline mortality frequently these days and found myself depressed at having to think about end-of-life issues in the musical world as well.

After initially counseling me to discard the stately old Stieff and buy a newer instrument, our piano tuner, Bruce Anderson, had a second thought. We could attempt to glue the pins in, he suggested. He noted that he wasn't sure this method would work but deemed it worth trying.

Bruce is a busy guy so he wasn't able to work on the pins until two weeks ago, when he arrived with a bottle of pin glue and a fold-up aluminum dolly. He used the dolly to lay the piano on its back and remove the keys and the action. He then applied the glue to the pins. Bruce explained that the piano had to remain at bed rest for a week and a half. At the end of that time he promised to return and see whether the thing could be tuned.

The week and a half were suspenseful—and not a little awkward. We had had to move furniture and rugs to accommodate the Stieff's wider-and-longer-than-usual footprint.

When Bruce returned, I was apprehensive. I always try to be optimistic. Nevertheless, in this case I feared that I would soon feel a bit like Bette Davis in *Dark Victory*.

Classic-film lovers will recall that for part of the film Davis's character doesn't know she has an inoperable brain tumor since her doctor (also her sweetheart, played by George Brent) lies about it to keep up her spirits. One day, however, she chances upon her file on his desk—and there in bold letters she reads the ominous words "Prognosis Negative."

As Taffy and I watched Bruce stand the Stieff back on its feet and rummage through his tuning equipment, I was concerned that we might hear those words (or something like them) from him.

Within a few minutes, however, our fears were dispelled.

On Bruce's last visit he hadn't been able to tune the piano at all. It was soon clear that the pin glue had changed that situation.

We now have a tuned piano!

The tone is just as rich and bright as I remember. The wood in the soundboard still has a few cracks, but Bruce will bring us a humidifier soon to keep them from getting worse.

"I'm glad you saved this piano," he said as he finished up tuning and gave Taffy a chance to run her fingers over the keyboard. He was the one who saved it, and I'm hugely grateful.

"It sounds lovely," Bruce added. "And I like to see old things get their lives extended."

Of course, I concurred.

Thursday, April 14: Upside Down

We ARE alive in the Weisblat household this week; we're just a little confused. Here's a brief rundown. It will HAVE to be brief because the Tinky laptop is on the fritz and so I cannot use it to type. The laptop will be shipped to IBM for repairs within the next day or so. At least, I hope it will.

Also on the fritz is poor Lorelei Lee. Our cat is throwing up on rugs, floors, and (you guessed it!) bedding. Her vet says the medicine we have ought to take care of the problem within a few days—if my fingers survive that long without major injury.

(I am good at holding down her paws as I pop pills into her mouth, but it's hard to avoid those sharp Siamese teeth when my fingers are right next to them.)

The good news is that Taffy seems to be doing reasonably well. True, she has a night or two of sleeplessness every week (her bad nights tend NOT to coincide with Lorelei's). And every once in a while she gets a little ornery.

Nevertheless, she is relatively perky and happy most of the time and has even begun to watch a little television with me of an evening. This is relatively recent as she has trouble with narrative. She is particularly fond of old variety shows. And she adored the first installment of the new *Upstairs Downstairs*.

So we are muddling through. I hope to write more words more brilliantly when the laptop returns to health.

Tuesday, April 19: Why I Dyed My Hair

I deluded myself in recent weeks that the little (okay, maybe not so little) gray patch at my temple looked more or less blonde in most light.

Now, however, I sport nothing but brown locks—the shade L'Oreal calls "Truffle," appropriately since Truffle is my dog's name. Here's the story.

Last Thursday I had ONE OF THOSE DAYS. It was a challenge to find good news to balance all the bad news. But I managed … until the end of the day, when one of my worst fears was realized.

The day began at my brother's house, where David kindly entered my financial information into his income-tax software.

The bad news there: despite having three different businesses I made a pathetically small amount of money last year. The good news: the government owes me money!

When I returned home, I found (good news) that UPS had delivered the box in which I was to send my sick laptop to IBM.

Bad news: the natives in our house were restless. Neither my mother nor my dog took to the idea of waiting around in the apartment for the scheduled pickup of the laptop in said box.

Taffy, who turns out to have one of her recurring urinary-tract infections, was at her most restless, insisting that we didn't have to stay home for the UPS man but could intercept him on the road if we went for a drive.

She made frequent forays to the door (which I had chained) to try to open it and yell for help from passersby. I tried gentle conversation, music, and a snack. She was adamant.

Truffle, hearing the door open over and over again (and hearing me explain repeatedly to my mother that someone was coming soon), began to bark incessantly.

Eventually, my mother settled down reluctantly. The dog went into her crate, where she tends to be quiet. Our cat Lorelei began to show signs of hunger so I decided to give her some stomach medicine, which she is supposed to take an hour before eating.

Between the noise and general grumpiness, her highness was NOT in the mood to be fed a pill. I wrapped her in a sweater and opened her mouth.

She promptly sprayed me. Urine seemed to flow everywhere— onto the furniture, my clothing, my face.

The good news here is that we do have a washer and dryer, not to mention good old soap and water. Eventually, the UPS man came, my mother and Truffle had a lovely ride in the car, and Lorelei's vet prescribed medical cat treats to take the place of the pills.

The custom-made treats are horrendously expensive. I would rather skimp on any number of luxuries, however, than try to feed this cat another pill. Ever.

One last piece of bad news lay in wait for me. We passed the doughnut shop on our ride, and I asked my mother if she would like me to buy her something special for breakfast the next day. Sweet lover that she now is, she assented happily. She and Truffle stayed in the car while I ran into the store.

Good news: I was thrilled when the nice young man behind the counter gave me a discount on the doughnuts.

Bad news: I was devastated when I looked at my receipt and realized that it was a SENIOR-CITIZEN discount!

Although many of my relatives call me cheap, my cheapness is exceeded—greatly exceeded—by my fear of aging.

Being seen as old to Tinky is like Moby Dick to Ahab, Waterloo to Napoleon, wire hangers to Joan Crawford, the capitalist oppressor to the proletariat, garlic to a vampire, Voldemort to Harry Potter, Christmas pudding to Oliver Cromwell, the Headless Horseman to Ichabod Crane....

I could go on, but I'm sure you get my drift.

Today I still have a sick mother (now on medication for her infection), an ornery cat, and a loud dog.

But by golly my hair is entirely brown.

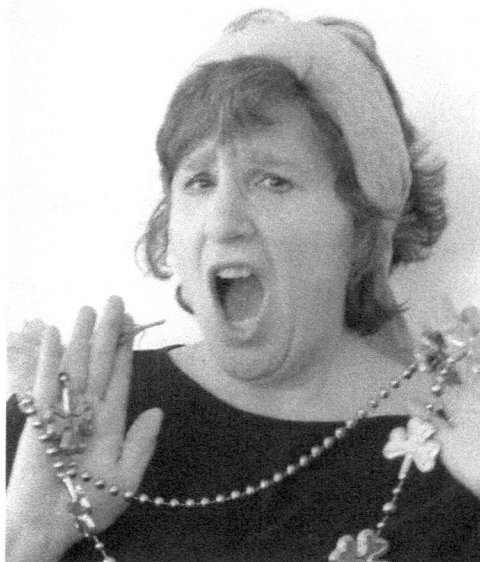

April Meditation: Mount Holyoke and Female Friendship

My mother's four years (1935-1939) at Mount Holyoke College in South Hadley, Massachusetts, formed her in many ways. The school gave her skills, confidence, and lifelong friendships.

Taffy decided that Mount Holyoke was her first-choice school after touring the campus in 1934. Her guide was Mary E. Tuttle, who would graduate in the Class of 1937. Taffy took to the outgoing, self-confident Tut and made up her mind to attend the college on the spot. Miss Tuttle was still active on campus when I got to Mount Holyoke several decades later. She never lost her zest for life or interest in fellow residents of the college.

Mount Holyoke was founded as a female seminary in 1837; Taffy was a student during the college's centennial year of 1937. A single-sex college, Mount Holyoke had (and still has) a history of turning out women who loved learning and social justice ... and who were strong in their belief in themselves and in sisterhood.

At Mount Holyoke Taffy continued her love of French, a language she had studied extensively in high school. She was proud that her connection with French (along with her lifelong love of dramatics) was alluded to in the book *On a New England Campus*, published in 1937.

Author Frances Lester Warner, who had visited the college for a year, wrote, "We never had a more bewitching performance than the recent acting of a certain freshman in tall pointed hat and white cotton wig as *Le Médecin* in Molière's play." That freshman was my mother.

The freshman's favorite French professor, Paul Saintonge, and his wife Connie adopted a few French students each year, and Taffy/Jan was among their adoptees when she arrived on campus in 1935. In 1936 the Saintonges took a group of students to France over summer vacation, and Jan fell irrevocably in love with the country. She would spend her junior year abroad there, studying at the Sorbonne and living with a French matron who found her American lodger unsophisticated but adorable. While in France Taffy became a social butterfly, flitting about a golden Europe on the cusp of world war.

Her skill with the French language also deepened from proficiency to knowledge during her time in Paris. "I learned that to speak excellent French was important, but that *what* I said was more important," she recalled later in life.

Taffy had always been smart, but in high school she had been a bit awkward. At Mount Holyoke she blossomed into a person who knew the value of her brain. And she developed friendships that would stand her in good stead all her life.

I can't list all of her college chums here, but I can tell you about a few. I was lucky enough to see them interact with Taffy first hand. I learned from each of them.

The friend who lasted longest wasn't actually a Mount Holyoke student but rather a young woman from another college who participated in the same junior-year-abroad program in France. Riley Moore was a native Washingtonian from an old Virginia family. She went on to marry an Uruguayan diplomat, Juan Yriart, and live in many corners of the world; Juan grew to be a great friend and colleague of my father. Riley was very chic and very proper, but she had a wonderful sense of humor. And she was one of the most supremely competent women I have ever known.

One of the things Riley and my mother had in common was marrying incredibly charming men. Luckily, they had enough confidence in their own intelligence and capacity for friendship to smile quietly (they were too well bred to roll their eyes) when many of the people they knew more or less ignored them and worshipped at the feet of their more outwardly impressive husbands.

The Yriarts ended up back in the Washington, D.C., area in retirement, allowing the friends many opportunities to see each other over the years. Riley died only a little more than a year before my mother. Despite my mother's dementia and Riley's infirmities, they treasured their visits together even at the end of their lives, although Riley had no illusions about either my mother or me. When we arrived half an hour past the appointed time for lunch one weekday, she announced, "I'm sorry to say this, Janice, but I told the staff you would be late!"

My mother laughed when she heard this, and after a startled moment Riley laughed with her. They had known each other for 70 years. They hardly had to speak in order to communicate.

My mother was a bridesmaid at Riley's wedding. She performed the same function for her friend Kay from Mount Holyoke. Katharine Irons looked like a movie star when she married Platt Brett in the early 1940s, and Platt always saw that young, beautiful bride when he looked at her throughout their long marriage. Kay was my godmother, and she took godmothering very seriously. I still treasure gifts and words she gave me.

Kay wasn't an easy person to be related to. She tended to hold grudges and had no idea how to be flexible. Yet she was a caring godmother to me and a loyal friend to my mother. They both enjoyed the world of words. Kay was the poet laureate of the state of Delaware. Her poems reveal a thoughtful, idealistic person.

I actually had two godmothers. My brother's godmother, another Mount Holyoke chum of my mother, decided that I should be her godchild as well and adopted me. Dagny Johnson (whom we called Dody) was an immensely charming woman with two loves in her life: France and the Florida Keys.

While she and my mother were on their junior year abroad in France Dody contracted polio. She never again walked without assistance. Yet she lived a remarkable life. She was named a Chevalier de la Légion d'Honneur by the French government in recognition of her work to preserve French films. A small park named after her near her home on Key Largo pays tribute to her efforts to sustain the ecosystem of the Florida Keys.

Being around Dody was an exhilarating and sometimes maddening experience. She had passion for—and a strong opinion about—everyone and everything she encountered. Her pronouncements were never simple statements; each sentence was filled with capital letters and ended with an exclamation point. Each vista she looked at, each mouthful she ate, was THE MOST WONDERFUL example of its kind—something to be savored and shared with friends.

One of Dody's greatest joys was the view she saw daily from her little house on Key Largo. Each afternoon she turned her sights and those of her guests to the coming sunset over the Gulf of Mexico. She argued it was best enjoyed sipping a cocktail or nibbling on a refreshing piece of key-lime pie. We were told to linger over the sunsets. No one could stop watching until the first star came out.

Like Dody herself those sunsets over the bay were colorful and dramatic. Like her they imposed their rhythm on those who came near them: they forced us to slow down and adapt to their pace. And they were always worth the trouble it took to drop whatever we were doing and yield to their appeal. I remember Dody whenever I see a sunset or taste a piece of key-lime pie.

My mother's last great friend from college was Sylvia. In 2009 I took Taffy to her 70th college reunion at Mount Holyoke. Watching the parade of alumnae—beginning with the Class of 1934 and ending with the Class of 2009—was inspiring. From the old ladies remembering their youth to the young girls looking ahead to their prime, these women in white exuded confidence, humor, and joy.

The college made a great fuss over the eldest alumnae at the reunion. Graduates officially return to the campus once every five years so the Classes of 1934 and 1939 were enjoying their moment in the sun. My mother particularly loved the hour or so we spent at the French department open house. There graduating seniors and returning alums mingled with faculty and staff. Taffy couldn't remember much French by then, but she loved hearing it spoken at the party. And she was thrilled to see two signs of her own time at Mount Holyoke on the wall of the French department library.

One was a plaque dedicated to her beloved professor Paul Saintonge. Above the plaque was a black-and-white photograph of a young woman wearing pearls. It bore a striking resemblance to my mother's own yearbook photo from Mount Holyoke. "My goodness," I said to Taffy, "that's Sylvia."

"Oh," responded my mother in the closest tone to a gush she could come up with (she was emphatically not a gusher), "MY SYLVIA!"

The subject of the photo was indeed her late friend Sylvia Delight Sherk Hubbell. Sylvia's family had established a memorial fund in her honor, and the college remembered her daily with this picture.

Sylvia lived up to her middle name and was a delight all her life. The daughter of missionaries (she led missionary children out of Iran at the onset of World War II), Sylvia wasn't the smartest or the most ambitious of my mother's friends. She was without a doubt the most adorable. She had a childlike enthusiasm for life that was infectious.

When she and my mother got together they were transformed into young girls. My mother would announce, "And now Sylvia Sherk will give her famous hog call," or, "And now Sylvia Sherk will stand on her head." Sylvia would comply, and they would both giggle. They probably didn't help each other learn a lot of French in college. But they obviously taught each other a lot about friendship. Sylvia, Riley, Kay, Dody, and Taffy taught me a lot about it as well.

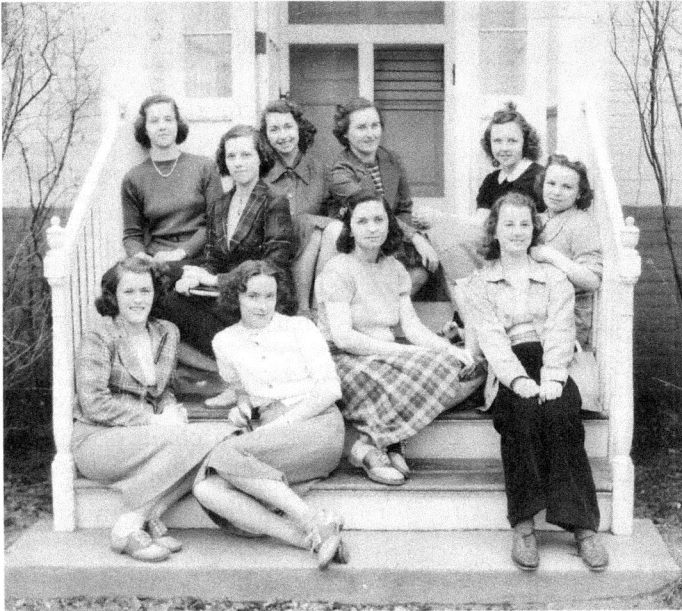

The residents of Mount Holyoke's French House, "Le Foyer," in 1939, with house president Jan Hallett on the far right

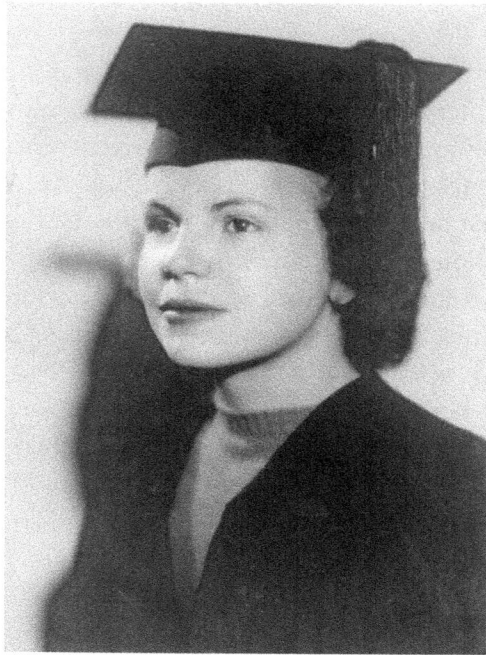

Taffy's graduation picture

Kay Brett wrote the poem that follows for Mount Holyoke's commencement in 1986. It sums up the ties my mother's generation of graduates felt to their past at Mount Holyoke. Mary Lyon was Mount Holyoke's founder. The bell that bears her name is in the college clock tower. It marks the quarter hours of each student's days and is always a welcome sound to alumnae returning for reunion. The laurel parade, in which seniors (dressed in white, like alums) march across the campus to leave a chain of laurel leaves on Mary Lyon's grave, is one of the highlights of each graduation weekend. The poem is reprinted here with the permission of the Brett family.

You, in Proud White Dress
by Katharine Irons Brett

This day belongs to you—
clean lakes, skies painful blue,
trees, walks, the "hi's"—
all intimately yours. All applies
to being a special part
of something so elusive
it's pictured only in the heart.
Please be aware it is inclusive,
for poignant memory
will never let the picture fade
for us who went before. We
once owned these green places.
Ours were the young, expectant faces;
ours now, the shadows lingering in the shade
Listening, watching the parade;
ours, the voices whispering through the leaves.
Have you not heard the echo purely
at chapel vespers as it weaves
its praise with yours? We are not dead
nor ever will be. As surely
as flows water ever fresh along the brook,
as surely young eyes eagerly will look
at these same walks and trees, will own
our lakes and books and buildings all,
will whoop at Mountain Day in fall,
will soak spring sun out on the lawn;
then dress in white as generations have,
make pilgrimage with laurel to a grave;
will listen to the call of Mary Lyon's bell
through growing, changing years sound, "All is well."

April Recipe: Key Largo Key Lime Pie

This pie always makes me think of my mother's college friend Dagny Johnson. To me it captures sunset in a pie shell.

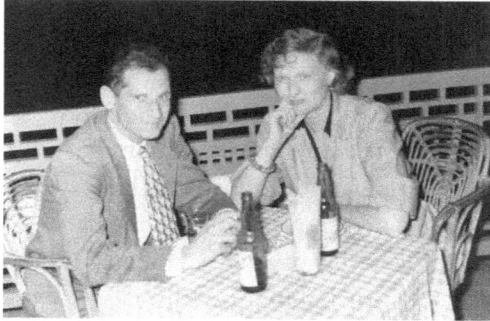

*The glamorous Dagny, with her friend Vince, in Cuba in 1950
(Courtesy of Eric Johnson)*

Ingredients:

1/2 cup key-lime juice

1 can (14 ounces) sweetened condensed milk

3 egg yolks (use the whites in another recipe; you won't need them here)

1 8-inch pie shell with a graham-cracker crust

whipped cream as needed

Instructions:

Preheat the oven to 350 degrees. In a medium bowl whisk together the juice, condensed milk, and egg yolks until they are smooth. Pour this mixture into your pie shell, and place the pie in the oven. Bake for 15 to 20 minutes.

The pie won't necessarily set, but you don't need it to!

After removing the pie from the oven let it cool to room temperature; then cover it and place it in the freezer until a few minutes before you are ready to eat. Remove the pie from the freezer, adorn it with whipped cream (either all the way across the top or just around the edges, depending on how much additional fat you want to absorb!), and serve. If you have leftover pie, store it, covered, in the freezer.

Serves 6 to 8.

MAY
Watching and Waiting
Sunday, May 1: Watching the Wedding

It took me a while to decide to watch the royal wedding on television.

I was torn at the prospect of the nuptials. I'm not a huge fan of royalty or of weddings, and I hate to get up early in the morning. On the other hand, I AM a huge fan of hats, and I like to keep my finger on the pulse of popular culture.

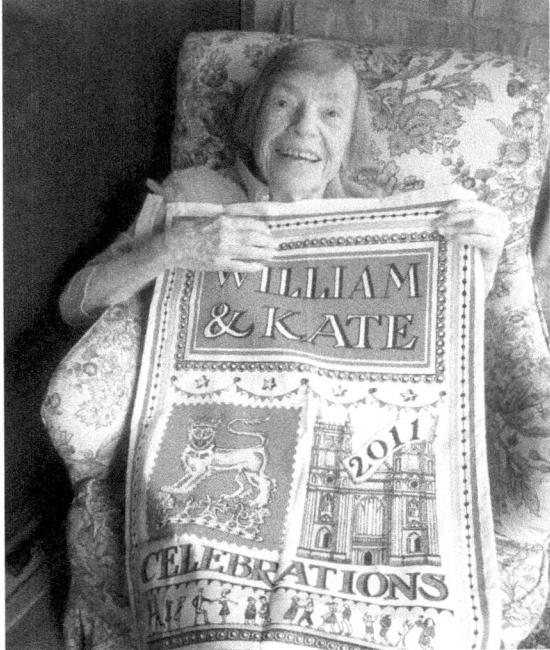

Two things tipped the scales toward watching.

First, my college roommate Kelly, now living in London, sent me a tea towel to celebrate the festivities.

I'm still using my Charles and Diana candy tin for food storage. I think the royal family is best enjoyed in memorabilia, although I don't go to the lengths of the enthusiast interviewed by John Oliver (who knows how to lace his contempt with just a touch of sympathy) last week on *The Daily Show with Jon Stewart*. The woman's collection included, among other bizarre items, bride-and-groom wedding gnomes for her garden.

So Kelly's gift gave me a warm feeling about the wedding.

The feeling grew warmer when I realized that I didn't have to get up at three in the morning to watch the beginning of BBC America's coverage, thanks to my handy-dandy DVR. I decided to give the wedding a whirl.

The event turned out to have a bonus I hadn't even considered when I set the DVR to record all 11-1/2 available hours (after all, I could always fast forward) of the BBC's wedding programming.

My mother was riveted by the whole thing.

I'm still trying to figure out precisely why.

She was never quite sure where it was taking place. (I think I must have had to tell her "Westminster Abbey in London" about 45 times as we watched the ceremony.)

She wasn't even certain who the principals were. When I pointed to the queen, she appeared to find the monarch familiar, although she did say "she's awfully old" several times. (Actually, I thought Elizabeth and the Duke of Edinburgh looked pretty good at 85 and 90.)

Prince William, Prince Harry, the bride, and the rest of the gang needed much more explanation. I didn't even bother with Elton John and Posh Spice. I found the latter's wedding attire too bleak to contemplate, anyway. Her black hat made her look like an angular bird.

Nevertheless, something about the day held Taffy's interest. Perhaps the universality of the ceremony and the events surrounding it struck a chord in her memory. She has never actually been to a wedding at which the streets were lined with well wishers. Nonetheless, she seems to share the perennial human interest in who wears what, who gets to the ceremony in what order, and what is said and done at a wedding.

Perhaps she just loved the color, spectacle, and music of the event.

The only segment that bored her was the Bishop of London's homily. (Sorry, Your Grace!) Unlike everything else that day, it was too wordy for her current cognitive level.

The homily aside, the wedding turned out to be the highlight of her week.

Now, if only Prince Harry would find the right girl and provide us with another royal show..........

Friday, May 6: Life's Little Luxuries

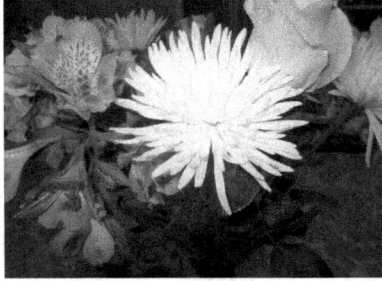

Life has been quiet on the Taffy/Tinky front lately, mainly because poor Taffy is now recovering from yet another infection.

We are going to the urologist on Tuesday in the hope that he can shed a little light on these recurring illnesses. Meanwhile, I'm trying to remain positive by counting our blessings, which are many.

Here are a few of them:

We have helpful friends and family members who call, write, think of us, and stop by. We just received a card from our church in Massachusetts. Its cover artwork was created by our minister. Cara is a talented artist as well as a sympathetic woman of the cloth.

For the past couple of days my mother and I have enjoyed extra friendship—a whirlwind visit (complete with fabulous belated Christmas presents) from our friend Peter. His dachshunds Lucca and Marco are Truffle's best friends in the world so our pooch had a special time as well.

We have competent, cheerful, and fun caregivers. Pertina and Brenda come by a few times a week to help out and give me a little time to run errands, work, or just take a nap.

My work is flexible so I can cut it back—often cut it out—when my mother is really ailing and needs special help.

We have the gift of music, which we listen to and make.

We have color all around us—on the plates from which we eat, in the paintings and hangings on the walls, even laced through the canopy that looms over our heads in the sunroom.

We are fortunate that Taffy has that rare thing nowadays—a pension. It pays for her care, for my health insurance, and for most of our household expenses, including the little luxuries that make her life and mine a pleasure.

Every time I walk into the house with a bouquet of flowers (about once a week), Taffy is enchanted. This week's arrangement, special for Mother's Day, includes roses that seem to send their aroma through the whole apartment.

We are working on the luxury of sleep. Meanwhile, we have just stocked up on French cheese, smoked salmon, and gorgeous fruit for Mother's Day, which we will celebrate with my brother David and his family.

Happy day to all the mothers, daughters, and sons out there—and to the animals.........

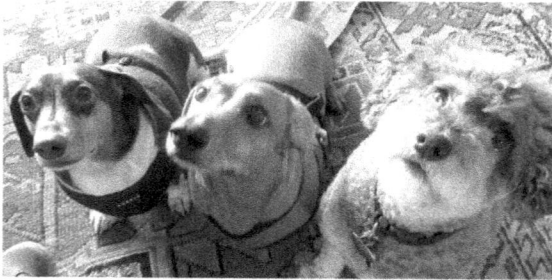

Thursday, May 12: A Quick Hospital Visit

As people age their relatives should expect more frequent visits to the hospital.

Nevertheless, my brother David and I were surprised to find ourselves sending Taffy to the emergency room last Saturday.

Whatever was wrong with her (and we're still not quite sure WHAT it was) came on very suddenly.

She slept in that day, ate a little breakfast, and settled down again for a nap.

When it came time to rouse her for lunch, however, I found myself unable to get her to stand up. I tried conversing and cajoling. She just closed her eyes a little more tightly.

I gave Taffy another hour or two to nap. When she was still unresponsive I called David. Together we attempted to get the mother upright.

We managed to help her stand. She couldn't remain standing, however, even with her walker, and she wasn't moving. Her demeanor was disconcerting and a bit scary.

So we called the EMTs.

We are still in northern Virginia, and I must say that visiting the emergency room here was quite different from my previous experiences. Those were in either very urban or very rural settings.

Both of those tended to be quite slow to help patients I brought in. In the city, gunshot victims and the like took priority. In the country, staff was minimal so everybody had to wait.

Here in the burbs—at least on this one day—the E.R. had room for everyone. Taffy was whisked in and immediately tested. The nurses and aides brought chairs into her little cubicle so David and I could keep her company and help with anything that was confusing.

The doctor knew all about patients like Taffy. As soon as she was tested and could walk again, thanks to the stimulation of the environment and the fluids the nurses had put into her veins, he released her.

He said that part of him wanted to keep her overnight for observation but the other part of him knew that she would be happier and less confused in her own home.

I am now trying even harder than before to make sure Taffy stays hydrated and has enough to eat. We think either low blood sugar or dehydration reduced her energy level. The doctor reminded me that many small meals work better than a few big ones for people who are reluctant to eat and drink.

Meanwhile, she is acting extremely perky. On Sunday she ate a hearty Mother's Day brunch. And her step is getting springier.

If—no, *when* (she is 92, after all!)—I have to take her back to the hospital I'll be a little less apprehensive about the process.

But I hope she waits a while to go.

Tuesday, May 17: Our Other Old Lady

More than one elderly female resides in our household. The lovely Lorelei Lee, our (mostly) Siamese cat, turned 20 a few days ago.

I'm suspicious of attempts to compare animal and human life spans so I won't tell you how old Lorelei is in feline years. But 20 is a significant age for her species.

She spent her birthday much as she spends many other days, although she was given extra special treats during the day—a morsel of pound cake here, a teaspoon of ice cream there.

Here was her basic schedule (which will be familiar to cat people).

Morning

Lounge in bed until forced out by cruel human who wants to wash the sheets.

Eat a few kibbles.

Use litter box, being careful to kick extra litter as far out of the box as possible.

Loiter in kitchen with large eyes until a shmear of cream cheese is deposited on a saucer on the floor.

Nap by self.

Noon

Hover at table during lunch begging for soup. Lap up soup.

Afternoon

Nap with Taffy.

Wake up and glare at vacuum cleaner.

Nap with Truffle (dogs make soft and warm napping companions).

Start yelling for dinner 1-1/2 hours before dinner time.

FINALLY eat dinner (baby food at this point in her life).

Use litter box, again kicking litter onto floor since previous litter has been cleaned up.

Nap by self.

Evening

Watch humans while they eat their dinner in the hope that a small amount of food will be placed on the floor.

Negotiate with the dog when said food finally reaches the floor.

Stand by water dish emoting until fresh water with crushed ice replaces the old water.

Nap with Truffle.

Eat a few more kibbles.

Get into bed. Groom Truffle and Tinky. Sleep.

Lessons Learned

As I said, this is a pretty typical day in Lorelei's life, although of course we don't change the sheets and vacuum every day.

Just as I learn from my mother, I learn from Lorelei Lee. She has many traits a person could do well to emulate. Here are a few of them:

First, the girl has admirable focus. I tend to get distracted. Once Lorelei Lee has decided it's time to do something she exerts all her energy to make it happen. I'm trying to cultivate that attitude.

She's also good at just letting go and relaxing; hence all the naps. I don't need to take several naps a day, but I would probably benefit from one or two, especially when Taffy hasn't been sleeping particularly well at night.

Lorelei is content with each of life's small pleasures—food, companionship, comfortable surroundings. Yet she knows how to stick up for herself when she thinks something (like the vacuum cleaner) is out of place. She strikes a good balance, one I'm still seeking.

And she is beautiful and impeccably groomed.

I'm sure I'll get there SOMEDAY. In the meanwhile, our elderly cat is a source of joy, amusement, and inspiration.

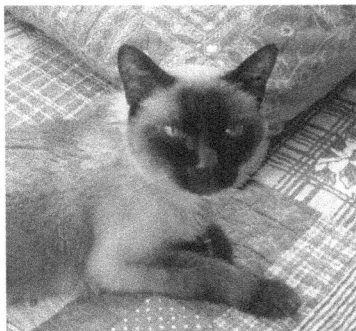

Friday, May 20: Sleep Talking

My mother has launched a new conversational pattern ... with herself.

A couple of days ago at the end of breakfast I asked her where she would like to go to sit, nap, and/or chat.

She said, "You go. I'll stay here. There is a lot to look at."

The dining room was indeed a busy space. Flowers, pill boxes, assorted cutlery, and a butter dish sat on the table.

Silver filled the sideboard.

And the plate rail sported its usual groupings of plates, pitchers, platters, vases, and figurines.

Taffy sat alone at the table for nearly an hour chattering to herself.

She generally appeared to be counting things although she never got further than five and she didn't always count in exact order.

She sang, "One, two, three O'Leary; three, four, five O'Leary; two, four, five O'Leary," as she pointed to imaginary items on the tablecloth.

Sometimes she veered into nonsense syllables. They didn't seem to be nonsense to her, of course, but I couldn't make them out.

At one point she reached down and picked one of Truffle's toys up from the floor. "You are five O'Leary," she told it and placed it next to the flowers on the table.

The entire exercise reminded me of talking in one's sleep.

Taffy's voice grew louder and softer as she conversed with herself. At her loudest and most assertive she had the plaintive resonance of a Lady Macbeth.

At her softest and most tentative she sounded more like a little girl talking to, and sorting, her toys.

Eventually she stood up and came into the living room where I was working. I asked her what she'd like to do, and she elected to listen to music. For a few minutes her arms waved in time as Fred Astaire, Rosemary Clooney, and Louis Armstrong serenaded her.

Eventually she went to sleep (but didn't talk).

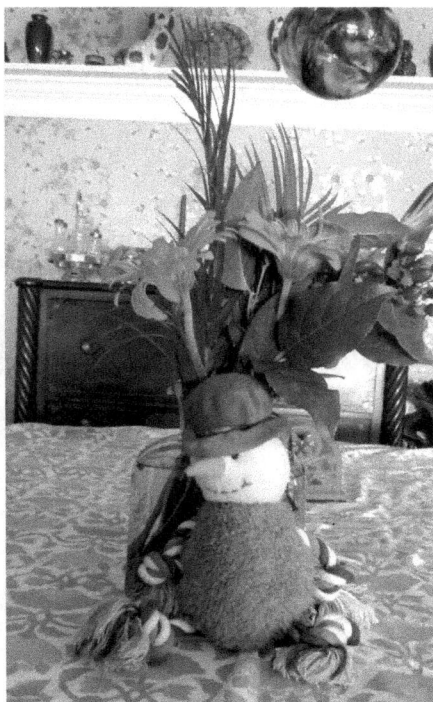

When she woke up, she was more herself, asking me questions about what we were going to do for the rest of the day. I have a feeling I haven't heard the last of her sleep talking, however.

I'm not sure what to make of this new phase of her dementia. In a way, her sleep talking is refreshing. When she is chattering on her own she has no need of entertainment. She is entirely self-sufficient.

On the other hand, it does seem to take her further and further away from the everyday world the rest of us experience. This might not be a bad thing for her peace of mind since she often has trouble understanding that world. It does concern me, however.

She was very much in the world for most of her life. Her disconnection from it may be a natural step, but it's a sobering one.

Friday, May 27: Music and Temperament

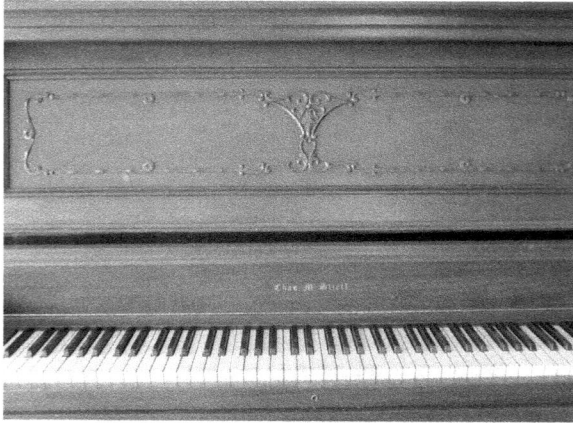

I have written before about the joy my mother takes in both listening to and making music.

Recently I read a book recommended by our piano tuner that brought the issue of my mother's relationship to music into focus (dare I say into tune?) a bit more.

The book is called *Temperament: the Idea That Solved Music's Greatest Riddle*. Published in 2001, it was written by a musician and historian named Stuart Isacoff.

The book revolves around a challenge in the history of music I hadn't known about before. I sing or play the piano daily, but my knowledge of music theory and history is purely practical. I've never studied either formally.

Isacoff writes that for centuries western civilization struggled with an odd mathematical incongruity in musical harmony. This incongruity became particularly obvious when the keyboard was invented.

Isacoff explains it a lot better than I can, but his basic point is that the proportions in string frequency that make up an octave (2 to 1) and a fifth (3 to 2) are incompatible. If one tunes a piano to create perfect octaves, one cannot tune it to create perfect fifths at the same time.

According to the author, the debate over how to tune pianos didn't involve only musicians. Philosophers, mathematicians, and even theologians cared deeply about trying to reconcile what were perceived as meaningful natural forms.

In the end, the then-controversial solution (still in use by tuners today) was to employ a technique called equal temperament, making the intervals on pianos ever so slightly different from the perfect proportions beloved of philosophers from Euclid on into the 18th century.

Isacoff is one of those authors who challenge the reader to think big. Even before he mentioned it in the book's final pages I was thinking of his work's relevance to string theory. This relatively new realm of physics suggests that the universe's most fundamental particles may be tiny strings that obtain their unique properties from their oscillation. (I know this sounds vague; I probably know even less about physics than I do about music theory.)

In addition to making me think about the history of philosophy and about nature of the universe, Isacoff also got me thinking about my own corner of the cosmos, my life with my mother.

Although she didn't grow up in an era in which music theory was seen as integral to our understanding of the universe and the nature of mankind, she did grow up in a time in which making music was a valued part of life.

She probably spent as many hours practicing the piano and singing around the house as she spent doing homework and thinking about "serious" academic subjects.

Although much of the book learning she acquired over a lifetime has abandoned her as her dementia has progressed, music still belongs to her. She relates to it with instinct, with knowledge, and with love.

In her brain and her heart music crosses over boundaries between past and present, between memory and forgetfulness.

I hope that future generations, who tend to consume rather than create music, can also retain a strong connection to musical forms as some of them age and lose memory—that they have the temperament to know and feel, as my mother does, that music is a cornerstone of humanity and of the universe.

May Meditation: The Owl and the Pussycat

A year after the events in this chapter—in May 2012—poetry lovers celebrated the 200th anniversary of the birth of author, poet, and artist Edward Lear. May 12 was named International Owl and Pussycat Day in honor of Lear's most famous poem, "The Owl and the Pussycat."

In my mother's house just about every day was Owl and Pussycat Day.

My mother never stood on her dignity. Indeed, dignity was not a word we used much to describe her. Instead she was playful, delighting in making silly faces and reciting nonsense verse.

She was always loved by small children, perhaps because a part of her never lost the wonder and fun of childhood. That sense of wonder and fun stood her in good stead later in life when her dementia brought her full circle to another form of childhood. She could always be distracted by a baby or a story or a song. And she loved to laugh.

In the meditation on her childhood I quoted her recollection of reciting "The Owl and the Pussycat" to anyone who would listen to her. She adored poetry so she also did a mean "Jabberwocky" and "Rice Pudding"—and even "The Boy Stood on the Burning Deck" and "Annabelle Lee." "The Owl and the Pussycat" was her signature poem, however, one that she recited all her life.

When I was a child and we attended neighborhood parties at Singing Brook Farm in Hawley, Massachusetts, her recitations were prominent features of our evenings. She was often slightly inebriated, but her voice never slurred.

Friends would pantomime the parts of the animals in the poem—the owl and the pussycat, who fell in love despite their obvious differences; the pig who sold them a ring for their wedding; the turkey who performed the marriage ceremony. And Taffy would loudly declaim the story, using all the melody in her voice and all the gestures in her short but sturdy body.

The trick with nonsense poetry, as Taffy well knew, is to recite it with a completely straight face. Each comical moment was spoken sympathetically. Each dramatic moment was spoken sincerely. She treated the nonsense/non-sense of the poem as complete sense, indeed as wisdom.

Thinking back on her many recitations, which merge into one in my memory, I now see that "The Owl and the Pussycat" was and is very wise indeed. It's a poem about the ways in which love is at once deathly serious and life-givingly silly. The owl and the pussycat fall in love and sail away "for a year and a day" to learn about each other and the world. The poem's lilting ending is enchanting:

And hand in hand, on the edge of the sand,
They danced by the light of the moon,
The moon,
The moon.
They danced by the light of the moon.

In her last couple of years Taffy and I would frequently recite the poem together. Not all of the words remained in her memory so I would feed them to her as needed. She always retained her sense of rhythm. And the poem continued to speak to her soul.

In an oddly comforting sense the poem represents our final year together to me.

Like the owl and the pussycat, we spent those months sailing toward the unknown and not always completely able to understand each other. Like them, we were also full of music (the owl loved to sing) and full of love.

In spirit we frequently danced by the light of the moon. In my memory Taffy dances by it still.

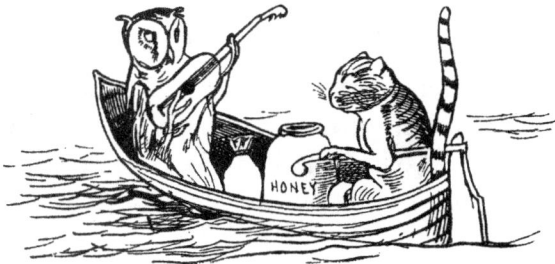

Edward Lear's sketch of the Owl and the Pussycat

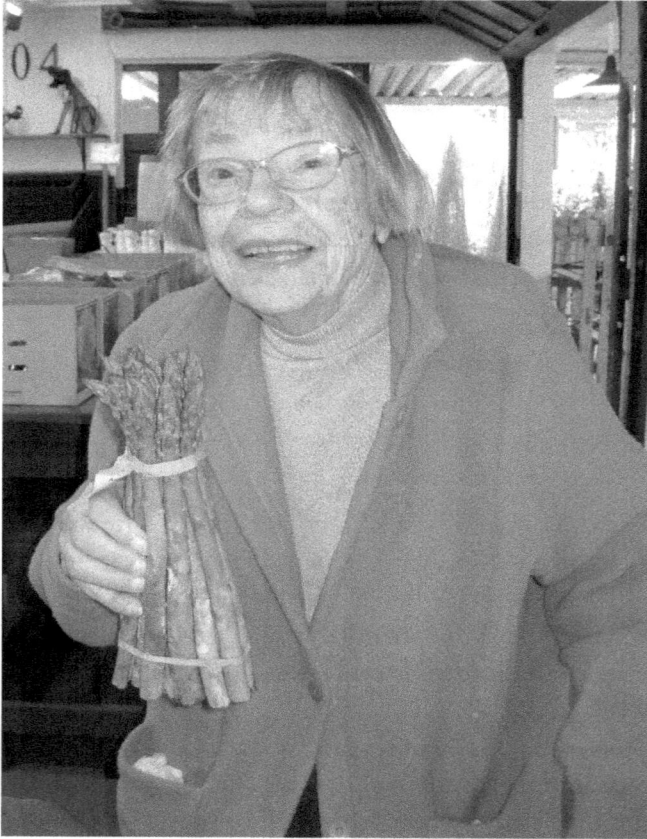

May Recipe: Green Emporium Asparagus Pizza

After writing about "The Owl and the Pussycat," I know I should probably feature a recipe that includes their favorite dishes, "mince and slices of quince." Those aren't exactly May foods, however, so instead I'm sharing a recipe based on a vegetable Taffy and I could have eaten every day during its May season, asparagus. The recipe comes from one of our favorite restaurants, the Green Emporium in Colrain, Massachusetts. The Green Emporium is now closed, but Taffy and I visited it frequently during her final years.

Ingredients:

1/2 to 1 pound asparagus (to taste)
1/2 cup extra-virgin olive oil plus 1/4 cup later
1/4 teaspoon red pepper flakes
1/2 cup grated Parmesan or Romano cheese (plus 3 to 4 tablespoons later)
1 teaspoon lime or lemon zest
1 teaspoon lime or lemon juice
1/4 teaspoon sea salt
1-1/2 pounds pizza dough
a sprinkling of cornmeal
1 heaping cup shredded mozzarella cheese, plus 1/4 cup later

Instructions:

Trim the bottoms off the asparagus spears, and cut them in thirds. Combine the 1/2 cup oil, red pepper flakes, 1/2 cup grated cheese, zest, juice, and sea salt. Toss in the cut asparagus spears, and let the mixture sit overnight.

The next day bring the pizza dough to room temperature and preheat the oven to 500 degrees. Place the dough on a round pan on which you have sprinkled cornmeal. Gently stretch the dough to a 16-inch diameter.

Using a brush or spatula, brush oil around the outer edge of the circle of dough; it should go from the very edge in about 1-1/2 to 2 inches. Sprinkle the heaping cup of mozzarella cheese evenly over the dough.

Place the marinated asparagus spears around the circle to resemble spokes of a wheel or a pinwheel design. The idea, according to Chef Michael Collins, is that "each piece [of pizza] will get more than its share of asparagus. You want it a little bit rustique."

Sprinkle the remaining mozzarella on top, "cementing the asparagus in." Follow with the remaining grated cheese.

Bake the pizza for 10 to 12 minutes, or until it is crispy and bubbly. (Cooks who have made pizza with tomato sauce will be surprised at how quickly this dryer pizza bakes, Michael notes.)

Let the pizza rest for a few minutes before slicing and eating. Serves 8 as a main course or 16 as a first course.

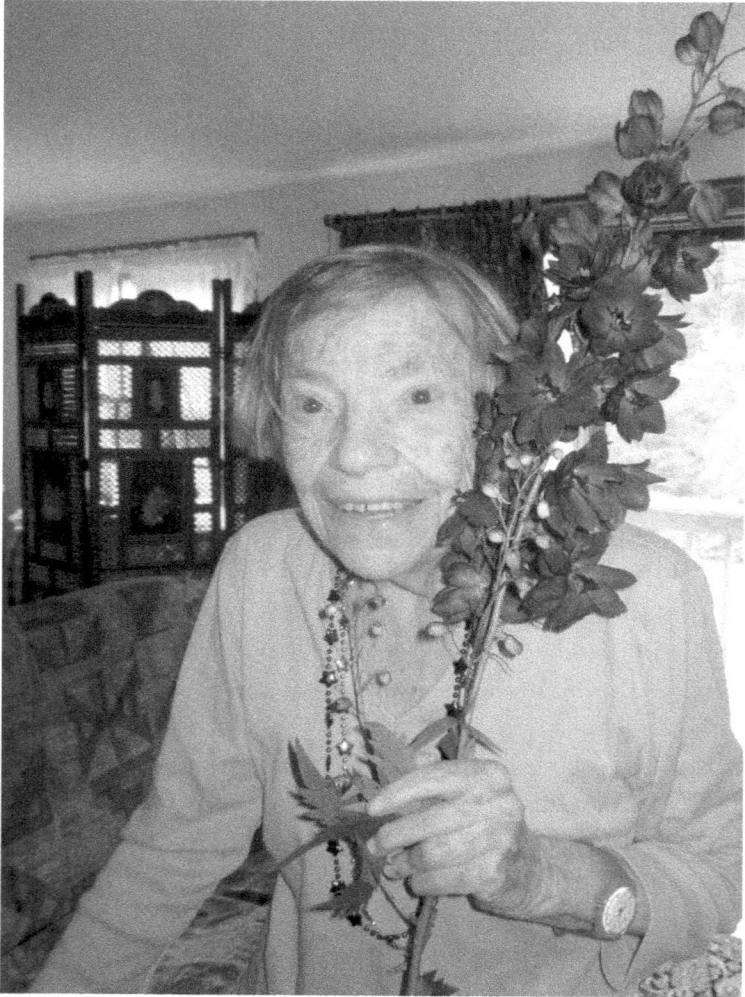

JUNE
The Road Home

Monday, June 6: Uncertainty

I haven't written much here lately. I have been waiting to determine the status of my mother's health.

A couple of days ago I realized that I should probably go ahead and write at least a few lines since I don't think I'm going to have a clear answer on that status for some time.

She has undergone all sorts of tests (none of them fun for her AT ALL) to try to nail down the source of the pesky white blood cells in her urine, without much luck so far.

In general, this is good news since one possibility was cancer of the bladder, which we know she definitely does not have. Nevertheless, I'm still longing for a bit more information.

She is definitely not thriving. Her appetite is diminishing. She is having trouble walking. And some days it takes a lot of time and effort just to get her out of bed in the morning.

This may just be the way she's going to be from now on. In that case, we'll have to increase caregiver visits or put her in an extended-care facility since she is becoming increasingly difficult for me to manage alone.

I hope that someone or something out there can help her.

We have yet another doctor's appointment this coming Friday.

The uncertainty is made more stressful for both of us by our desire to go home. My mother pleads to go home with increasing frequency. I empathize since I long for my own childhood home in Massachusetts (where we still have a house) as she longs for hers in New Jersey. I originally planned that we would return to Massachusetts in April.

We would both love to see the lupines and the rhododendrons there. (We've missed the daffodils and the apple blossoms this year, I'm afraid.)

It's a long trip, however, and I want to make sure she can manage it.

So I bide my time, plan writing projects, practice my singing, and swim whenever I can.

Taffy still enjoys time with family when she's awake. And she generally still appreciates music. She came to the program of Civil War songs our local music club performed yesterday.

We almost didn't make it to the performance since it took me so long to get her into the main passenger elevator of our building that the darn machine broke down, closed the doors, and refused to budge.

Otis calls the tendency of the elevators to stop working when the doors have been blocked a safety feature. I call it annoying.

We were trapped inside the stationary elevator for several minutes before the doors deigned to open. (Maybe it was only two minutes, but it felt like at least 15.)

Luckily, the building's service elevator was more forgiving. We finally made it out of the building and arrived at our destination just as the concert was due to begin. Taffy adored sitting in the audience with my brother. (Thank you, David!) She sang along in spurts and focused a lot of attention on a service poodle guarding its human companion nearby.

(I have a feeling she would like to get Truffle an ensemble with the words "service dog" embroidered on the back so the pooch could go everywhere with us.)

As for me, I sang with a big smile on my face. The music club had planned the program to accommodate my schedule since I was the only soprano who could hit the high B-flat at the end of "The Battle Hymn of the Republic," our grand finale. I was happy not to let my fellow musicians down.

Besides, I loved nailing that B-flat. We sopranos are a little vain about our high notes.

Such occasions are good for both my mother and me at times like this when the future seems so very foggy.

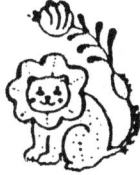

Thursday, June 9: Maudlin for a Moment

I try to avoid being maudlin except when singing sad songs on Saint Patrick's Day.

Tuesday evening I gave in to a maudlin mood, however.

It had been a long day with Taffy. I got her out of bed with great difficulty at 10:30 in the morning. She ate small meals but didn't really focus on much.

Late in the day she began talking to me, quite passionately, about the joys of school vacations.

I'm not 100 percent sure that was her topic, but I think it was. She wasn't very clear. She did seem to be talking about the weather, however, and what children like to do in their free months.

It reminded me of one of her favorite themes when she was still making more coherent conversation. She was wont to say that today's children are overscheduled, that they need time to spend lying on the grass gazing at clouds more than they need camp sessions or violin lessons or play dates.

Unfortunately, that reminder only served to make me realize how far her capacity to converse had deteriorated. On the surface I was happy to see her chattering away and tried to feed her good responses. Inside all I could do was echo one of her frequent requests.

Like Taffy, I WANTED MY MOTHER.

I decided it might cheer me up to list a few of the special qualities she exhibited over the years. Here they are, in no particular order.

She excelled at crossword puzzles.

She could cook for a crowd on a moment's notice; she particularly specialized in what she called "funeral baked meats."

She was cheerful.

She loved to learn about new people and places.

She recited poetry with elegance and eloquence, particularly silly verse like "The Pobble Who Has No Toes."

She offered quiet comfort when one was sad or sick.

She wrote and edited swiftly and skillfully.

She remembered people she hadn't seen in years and songs she hadn't heard in decades.

She had an unerring sense of direction.

She had an ear for languages.

She loved to laugh, dress up, and act.

She was loyal to old friends; to old neighborhoods; and to her alma mater, *Mount Holyoke College.*

She was stubborn to a fault. She, not unnaturally, thought of herself as "strong minded."

She expected excellence from my brother and me.

She took responsibility for mistakes and apologized if an apology was warranted. Yet she never felt guilt; she excelled at putting her mistakes behind her.

Her temperament and intelligence perfectly complemented those of my father. Together my parents showed their children different ways in which one could be smart, express affection, and cultivate friends.

That's as far as I got on the list before I realized that I still have a lot of the mother I was describing.

Some of the qualities she still has herself. She is often still loyal and interested in people, particularly children. Her level of cheerfulness has diminished, but it hasn't completely disappeared. Heaven only knows, she is still stubborn.

Some of the qualities reside in my brother, including the sense of direction (NOT something I ever absorbed), the vivid memory, and the loyalty.

And some I have inherited. I certainly love to laugh, dress up, and act. And I'm afraid that I, too, am "strong minded" to a fault.

I wish I could say that either of Taffy's offspring had inherited her freedom from guilt. I'm afraid that recessive Protestant trait was cancelled out by our father's Jewish genes.

I'm thinking of trying crossword puzzles to see whether I can cultivate that skill. Meanwhile, my maudlin moment has passed.

Wednesday, June 15: Kind of Sort of Better ... by Accident

Life with an elderly person is full of surprises.

My last couple of journal entries noted that my mother was ailing of late.

I wouldn't say that she is thriving at this point. She's definitely quite a bit better, however.

For most of last week she slept for a lot of the day. When she wasn't sleeping she was unhappy about much of life and uncharacteristically hard to cheer up.

One morning she suddenly changed. Instead of seeing a sleepy, nervous death's head when I popped into her room to check on her I saw a smiling face—and a body that was on the move. It wasn't moving fast, but it was moving.

She has continued to appear reasonably strong. She can't walk far, but her gait is much improved. And she is having fun again. A couple of days ago my brother and I took her to a nearby pool, along with five 11-year-old youngsters. She didn't swim, but she took great pleasure in chatting and napping near the water and in watching the children frolic.

Every silver lining has a tiny cloud. Since Taffy hasn't been particularly mobile recently I have relaxed my vigilance about chaining the front door of our apartment shut.

Yesterday as I was assembling the maternal breakfast in the kitchen she hoofed it over to the door with her walker and made her escape into the hallway.

Thanks to the sudden heated barking of our watchful dog, I caught Taffy before she made it into the elevator and out of the building. Apparently, Truffle knows that her mom isn't supposed to take unauthorized solitary excursions. I'm thinking of renaming our smart little canine "Lassie."

Despite this momentary dilemma I don't worry overmuch about the risks of Taffy's improvement. I can chain the door. I can't infuse her with artificial perkiness.

I'm still not super bright about medical stuff, but I'm learning. I think I have found the cause of my mother's improved gait and alertness.

She recently had a tooth taken out. (Unfortunately, her teeth, which lasted valiantly for 85-plus years, are finally leaving her.) The dentist prescribed antibiotics to prevent her mouth from becoming infected as it healed.

A few days later she exhibited the sudden signs of renewed health.

We saw Taffy's primary-care physician on Friday. She wasn't sure why Taffy was so down before or why she responded so well to the drugs. Dr. Carter didn't doubt the response, however. Unfortunately, Taffy has been scheduled for yet another test later this week ... so we won't be able to go home to Massachusetts until at least the end of next week.

I'm keeping my fingers crossed that my mother will still be feeling relatively energetic then.

Meanwhile, we're trying to squeeze as much enjoyment as we can out of life. The table offers Taffy an array of treats. We go for short rides in the car and shorter walks with the dog.

And we make lots and lots of music.

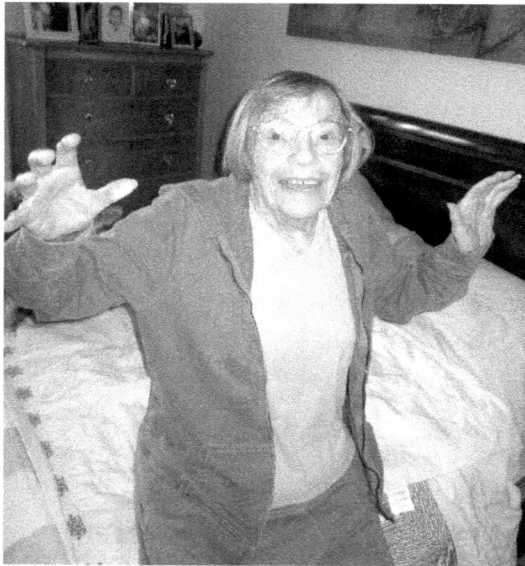

Taffy on the mend

Tuesday, June 21: Sorrow and Gladness

My neighbor Alice Parker composed a haunting choral piece called "Sorrow and Gladness" with lyrics by Gracia Grindal. Grindal adapted the words from a 17th-century text.

The song begins,

Sorrow and gladness are sister and brother,
Fortune, misfortune, both stand side by side....

That mingling of sorrow and gladness, laughter and tears, characterizes all of life. Lately I have been struck particularly by the ways in which it sums up my current journey with my mother.

Good news and bad news each enjoyed a day with us this past weekend.

Saturday was our bad-news day.

Taffy generally shows little awareness of her memory loss. Saturday saw the exception to that rule.

She gazed at the photographs of her parents in her room, ordinarily a source of joy and solace for her. Suddenly, however, she told me that she couldn't remember their names or anything about them.

Over and over I repeated her mother's and father's names and recounted their life stories as she had told them to me (and as I had eventually observed them myself).

She refused to be comforted, mostly because in her current state the information blew out of her head as soon as it blew in.

Eventually, I suggested that I practice music. My singing usually makes her happy. She waves her hands, hums, and sometimes even sings lyrics.

Saturday it didn't work. She covered her ears when I started vocalizing. She was particularly upset by the song "'Murder,' He Says," a comedy number by Jimmy McHugh and Frank Loesser. Its singer complains about her boyfriend's inappropriate language during intimate moments. The main line goes, "He says, 'Murder,' he says, every time we kiss."

"STOP TALKING ABOUT MURDER!" shouted my mother. "I don't want any murder in here." And she cried and cried.

Eventually, my brother came to dinner. His company, plus the dog and some Indian food, cheered Taffy up.

In fact, it was an idea of my brother's that made Sunday a success. He suggested that I try watching the U.S. Open golf tournament with our mother, pointing out that it had no narrative to confuse her.

Sure enough, when I turned the television on Sunday afternoon she was riveted. When we talked or did something while waiting for the golf to resume—she helped me administer medicine to the cat, for example—Taffy spoke like a rational adult rather than the frightened child she had seemed the day before.

Part of me wishes we could watch golf every day. Another part of me realizes that it wouldn't work for her every day. Still, I'm glad gladness came through to displace its sibling for at least a while.

Wednesday, June 29: There's No Place Like Home

As I type this I'm looking out an open window through the bushes onto a serenely blue New England sky. After months of thinking we *might* be able to travel soon my mother and I are finally in residence at our home in Hawley, Massachusetts.

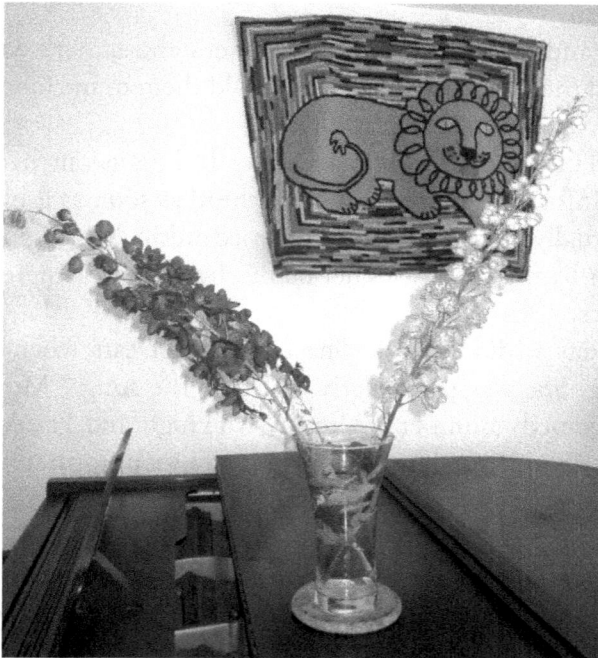

We drove up from Virginia on Saturday. The trip itself was an illustration of the ups and downs of life with dementia, with a little feline vomiting and a lot of traffic thrown in to spice things up.

Sorrow and gladness mingled once more on our journey: the worst part of the day was followed by the best.

The trip's nadir came when we crossed the George Washington Bridge from New Jersey into New York.

My mother had been alert enough to judge from the road signs that we were driving through New Jersey, her childhood home. When we left the state she became very upset and demanded that I take her back immediately to her mother's house in Maplewood.

For the next hour or so she was inconsolable. I seriously considered moving her to the back seat (where the door locks are childproof) in case she took it into her head to fling herself out of the car.

Unfortunately, that seat was crowded with the dog, food, shoes, and upholstery fabric. I held my breath and comforted myself with the knowledge that it takes her a while to unsnap her seat belt. Luckily, she stayed where she was.

After an extended period of screaming and crying we came to a stretch of road in New York State with which she was familiar. She had traveled along the Taconic State Parkway many times on the journey from her New Jersey home to New England.

Suddenly, the landscape delighted her. "This trip fills me with joy," she told me. "Thank you for bringing me."

She didn't recognize the house in Massachusetts consciously, but her body knows it. She has no trouble sleeping in her own bed at night and finding her way from her room to the bathroom. She is still tired from the long journey, but when she is awake she is mostly happy.

Sunday night we went with our neighbor Alice to eat pizza at our beloved Green Emporium Restaurant in Colrain, the frequent site of my chanteusification (next performance: August 27). Mike and Tony, the hosts, greeted Taffy with beaming faces.

Every day someone seems to stop in to say hello.

Yesterday was a particular highlight. Taffy's new friend and caregiver, Pam, came by to keep her company while I got the car inspected and so forth. They hit it off wonderfully; I returned home to the sound of soft laughter.

At the end of the afternoon, Taffy, Alice, and I went to Wilder Brook Farm to pick up our farm shares.

Possibly my favorite part of the share at Wilder Brook is the bouquet of flowers we receive each week. This week the highlight of the floral offerings was a group of spectacular delphiniums. (Delphinia? You know what I mean.)

Taffy stayed in the car while Alice and I went to get the flowers and vegetables. When we returned with full arms we discovered that Cheryl from our church had brought my mother a huge, deep purple delphinium.

On the drive home she enthused over it. "This is the most beautiful thing I ever saw," she exclaimed. "I don't know what I have done to deserve this lovely flower."

That evening at bedtime, as she frequently does, she told me it was time for her to go home.

"We ARE home," I replied (as I always do). "This house belongs to us."

"Really? To you and me?" asked Taffy.

"Absolutely."

She smiled a huge smile.

This morning she called for her mother again. A few minutes later, however, she was alert and ready to go buy strawberries with me. On the way home in the car she held the dog on her lap.

She whispered to Truffle, "We're on our way back up the hill to our favorite place in the whole world."

That whisper, the lush greenery everywhere, and the strawberries made me feel at home, too.

June Meditation: Taffy's Marriage

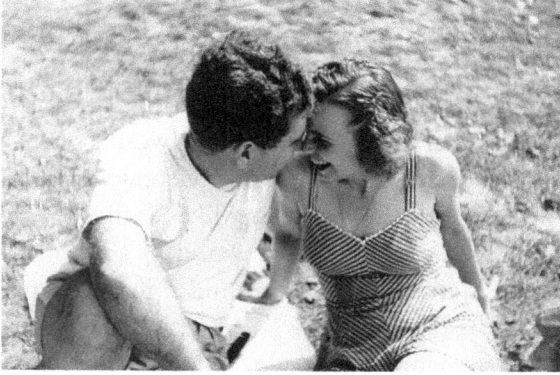

Taffy met my father when she went to work as an apprentice teacher in the elementary school at Stevens Hoboken Academy in 1941. A female colleague pointed out all the single male teachers to young Jan Hallett on her first day of work at the school. When her glance alit on the sixth-grade social-studies teacher and school librarian, Abe Weisblat, her fate was sealed.

The two fell in love quickly, and Jan wrote a series of poems to Abe. He later bound them into a book called *Blue Skies over Hoboken*. I would love to be able to share a poem or two with you, but at some point the book disappeared.

My brother and I do still have a scrapbook Taffy kept about their courtship. Most of its contents are programs from plays they attended and train-ticket stubs from her journeys to visit him once he left Hoboken to go to graduate school in Wisconsin.

There are a few notes from Abe, however. These show that he was a smitten as Jan was—and that he could be silly, a trait she cherished.

In a note from 1941 (it is dated only with the time, 6:30 p.m.) he wrote:

Dear Janice,

Since you feel you can trust me, I guess I might as well come to the point at once—How about a date for Saturday night at which I could save some money? As your Yale pal would say why spend money on the trimmings—can't we just go riding and parking?....

P.S. Don't feel too disillusioned—it happens over and over.

Early on Jan and Abe established a pattern of conflict resolution that lasted for most of their life together.

Jan suggested that since the two were in love they should get married.

"Oh, no," replied Abe glumly. He worried that since she was Christian and he was Jewish the marriage would never work.

I don't know what Jan's exact words were when he told her this, but it's very likely she said something like "Piffle."

Every time they got together for months she would argue that they should get married—and he would sigh and explain that the marriage would be doomed.

Eventually, she wore him down.

On June 24, 1944, at 4:42 (whether it was a.m. or p.m. is not clear!) he wrote:

My dear,

 This is to reply to your question: "Do I desire a million dollars more than keeping one Janice?"

 After careful deliberation and much thought I have come to the following conclusions:

 1. *I would not trade you for a million dollars.*
 2. *I love you.*
 3. *I want to marry you.*

Sincerely yours,

Abraham M. Weisblat

The couple still faced the task of convincing their parents that the match would endure. Both sets of parents liked their prospective in-laws, but neither set could envision its child marrying someone of another religion.

This may not seem like a major issue in the 21st century, but in the 1940s a Christian marrying a Jew or vice versa was a very big deal. The Weisblats wondered how Abe would feel the first time Jan called him a dirty Jew. The Halletts wondered how the young couple would bear not being able to join my grandfather's beloved Maplewood Country Club, which refused to accept Jewish members.

The parents asked them to remain engaged for a year to make sure the relationship would stick. At the end of the year, they were married twice (once in a Unitarian church, once by a rabbi). And the relationship certainly stuck.

Once they were married, Jan suggested they have children. "Oh, no," said Abe again, concerned that the children of such a union would grow up confused at best and discriminated against at worst.

So once again his beloved set to work on him. It took her seven years, but eventually he gave in. She threw away her diaphragm, and my brother was born nine months later. She later referred to Baby David as her "own personal miracle." I came along a few years after that. I may not have been a miracle, but I was loved!

I gather that my parents' early life together was punctuated by gigantic fights. In later years Taffy recalled throwing a camera at Abe at one point. By the time we children came along, however, they had worked out the kinks in their relationship.

His tendency to arrive early for every appointment had been tempered by her tendency to be late so that they were pretty much always on time. His occasional bouts of depression were buoyed by her relentless cheerfulness. They made friends together, entertained together, and divided up childrearing responsibilities efficiently. (She was the disciplinarian!)

They were fun and funny and smart in complementary ways. She was good with words, and he was good with people. In their prime they were an amazing team. They spent a lot of time apart because my father traveled extensively for work. Their separations made each of them stronger individually—and made them value each other's company more when they were together. Above all, they absolutely trusted each other in all aspects of life.

They were partners in my father's professional life as an agricultural economist working with people from developing countries. Such partnerships were not uncommon in their generation, particularly in the 1950s. Jan was Abe's hostess, his sounding board, his editor, and his primary adviser when it came to work.

The organization for which he worked for much of his career, a tiny Rockefeller-funded foundation known as the Agricultural Development Council, recognized the role of spouses in its employees' careers. Taffy frequently attended A.D.C. conferences and sat in on decision-making sessions. She also traveled with my father overseas every few years when he took off for a two- or three-month jaunt. (My brother and I stayed home in the States with relatives.)

Her participation in his professional life, and the travel it entailed, had a two-fold influence on their life together. First, it gave them a lifestyle they would never have been able to replicate if they had been traveling on their own dime. They stayed at first-class hotels around the world, and they had clothes and jewelry custom made in Hong Kong and elsewhere.

More importantly, the rhythm of that life made it different from the typical professional life of the 21st century; one could argue that the rhythm made the life more meaningful. My father and mother meandered from country to country on these trips, spending several days in most places. Their business contacts were cultivated not just at official meetings but at dinner parties and during sight-seeing excursions. They really got to know people with whom my father might be doing business—and in doing so established a level of trust and friendship that purely "professional" relationships don't always manage to forge.

Here's an example of how it all worked: In my mother's 1960 travel diary she discusses a trip the two took to Rome. They attended an audience with the Pope and had several meals and mini-trips with friends of friends in Rome and at the Vatican. It all sounds like pure tourism in her descriptions. There were no official meetings. There was no agenda—just a lot of sightseeing, conversation, and delicious Italian food.

I know, however, that four years later my father hosted a major conference about the role of the Catholic Church in the Philippines. He would never have been able to pull off the conference had he not gotten to know those people in Rome. He wasn't thinking of organizing such a conference when they met; he hadn't even yet been to the Philippines.

Nevertheless, by making new friends and letting conversations take their course, he and my mother established the conditions under which such a conference could be conceived of and organized.

It was a way of doing business that doesn't seem efficient at first glance but ends up becoming deeply efficient in the long run.

It was also a way of doing business that suited my parents perfectly. I have always thought of their marriage as one long dinner party. They loved dinner parties and threw them frequently. The food at the table was always good, and the conversation was never planned. At the end of the evening the participants felt nourished in many ways by this couple whose partnership was solid, strong, and just plain fun.

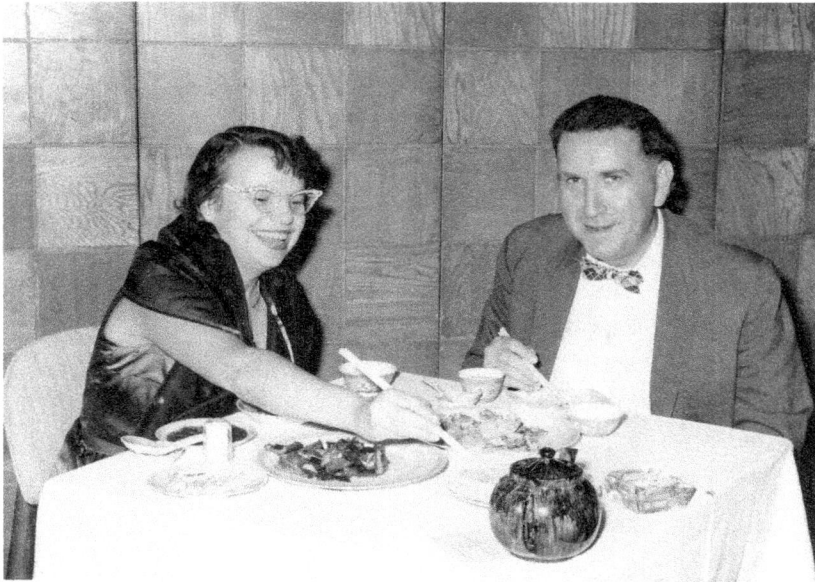

June Recipe: Green Goddess Dressing

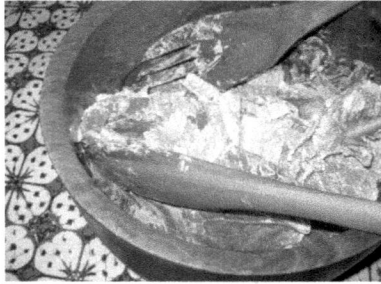

June is a month in which local salad greens are gloriously available. Taffy always enjoyed this dressing, based on one from my friend Donna Hill in California. And since June is the typical month for marriages I think salad is appropriate: Taffy's recipe for a good marriage was to mix things up, work a bit, and be positive. (It sounds rather like a salad, doesn't it?)

Ingredients:

1 clove garlic
4 anchovy fillets
1 scallion, chopped
1 generous tablespoon chopped fresh parsley
1 generous tablespoon chopped fresh chives
1 generous tablespoon fresh tarragon or basil
the juice of 1 lemon
2 cups of mayonnaise (homemade is best, but commercial—even low fat—is fine; just avoid fat free)
salt and pepper to taste

Instructions:

Place the garlic and the anchovy fillets in the bowl of a food processor and pulse until minced. Add the scallion, the herbs, and the lemon juice and process again; then add the mayonnaise, the salt, and the pepper. Process again until smooth.

Taste the dressing and adjust the seasonings accordingly.

Serve over a split romaine heart. (Or just shred some romaine, which works beautifully.) Garnish with a sprig of fresh basil or tarragon if you wish.

Makes about 2 cups of dressing.

JULY
A Golden Month

Tuesday, July 5: How Can I Keep from Singing

I apologize for the length of this essay! As we often do we have had our ups and downs this week in the Weisblat household. I've done snippets of writing here and there, and each time things went up or down I've had to add a bit to my chronicle. I'm afraid the narrative hasn't ended up entirely smooth—but then life isn't entirely smooth, either.

In general, the high spots of my time with Taffy this week have outweighed the low ones although they haven't canceled them out entirely.

Last Wednesday—shortly after I wrote here about my mother's sunny temperament and general feeling of being home, in fact—she took a turn for the worse.

Being attuned (finally!) to the signs, I took only a few hours to figure out that her symptoms indicated yet another urinary-tract infection. She was back on antibiotics by midday on Thursday.

It took her a long time to recover, however. She barely moved her feet for much of Friday. Indeed, she spent at least half an hour on the floor that morning. She had decided to sit down there for a rest, and it took quite a bit of persuasion and muscle (sometimes I literally pull Taffy) to get her onto a chair.

Luckily, music, friends, and antibiotics eventually perked her up. On Saturday and Sunday she was back in stride.

The turning point came Friday night. We had talked all week about going to the first concert in Mohawk Trail Concerts' summer season. We are lucky enough to be able to find chamber music ten minutes away from us, and Taffy has enjoyed the concerts since their beginning in 1970.

I was torn as the time to leave for the Charlemont Federated Church (home to MTC) approached Friday evening. On one hand, I knew that if we didn't go to the concert, Taffy wouldn't consciously miss it. And I didn't want to cross the line between stimulation and torture by dragging her to an event that would tire her out more than it would benefit her.

On the other hand, I knew that she loved music, particularly these concerts. And, let's face it, I was in the mood for a little chamber music myself!

So I worked hard to get her to the concert. We were actually a little late arriving because it took me so very long to transfer her from our couch to the wheelchair and thence to the car. I whisked the wheelchair into the church sanctuary just as co-artistic director Ruth Black was announcing the program.

An amazing thing happened when the concert started. In about ten minutes' time my mother moved from weak and listless to energetic and alert.

The music cut through her brain and went straight to her heart.

Of course, it's possible that the antibiotics chose that moment to kick in. Nevertheless, I credit much of her transformation to the power of that music. She stayed up until 10:30 that night and awoke refreshed the next morning, humming away.

On Saturday our neighbors at Singing Brook Farm organized their annual neighborhood Independence Day picnic by their Dam, a wonderful structure they fill every year so that the brave among us can enjoy an icy swim. As we nibbled we caught up with friends and neighbors—and watched Will Cosby and company put in the gate that traps water in the Dam.

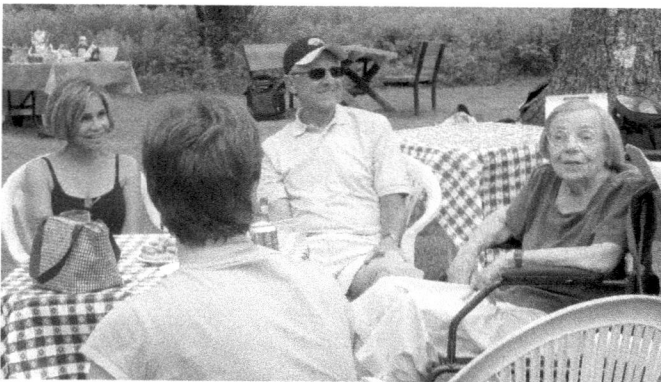

Taffy enjoys a convivial lunch at the Dam.

On Sunday the wonderful Pam gave us a few hours so she could bring Taffy to church to hear me sing all-American songs. Taffy enjoyed the company in church even more than the music. She was greeted by all and sundry with smiles and hugs. And our friend Susan brought baby Joshua to sit next to Taffy's wheelchair. My mother was mesmerized by the almost-one-year-old child; the two happily (and, luckily, QUIETLY) played through the service.

Sunday afternoon my cousins David and Mardi stopped by with their teenage children. My mother couldn't exactly identify any of the Smith clan (she took to calling young Brandon "Boy," which reminded me of nothing so much as Tarzan), but she clearly had a wonderful time visiting with them and enjoyed being taken out to dinner. "I don't know who those people are, but I really like them," she told me as they headed home to Connecticut.

By Monday the happy but busy weekend had tired Taffy out. When I let her take too long a morning nap to recover she ended up without enough food and drink in her system. It was all I could do to get her to sip a bit of energy drink from time to time.

Eventually the drink plus a little food revived her. We went down to the Dam. Taffy sat in her straw hat drinking in the sunshine and the greenery. I managed a foray into the frigid water to pay my respects to the mountain laurel on the far side of the Dam.

As I wheeled my mother to the car I remarked that our dog Truffle, who had retrieved her tennis ball from the water several times, seemed very happy.

"This is heaven for her," said Taffy. "For us, too. We will come here every day."

It was a lovely thought. Unfortunately, as my mother tried to get back into the house (we're working on a ramp, but for the moment we are stuck with a couple of unavoidable steps) she collapsed in a little heap. My neighbor Alice and her friend Jody helped me get Taffy into the house, feed her another very small snack, and settle her down for a nap.

She revived a bit later, but the weekend as a whole made me appreciate her increasing fragility even as it made me appreciate our friends, relatives, and neighbors.

I can't really regret packing so much activity into a few days. Taffy adored her holiday weekend. I do think we'll need to cut back a bit, however, since clearly fun has its price. As Taffy used to say in her more lucid days, taking "everything in moderation" is the key to happiness and health.

The ups and downs of our recent saga—and the role music has played in my mother's happier moments—remind me of one of the songs I sang in church Sunday morning, the Quaker tune "How Can I Keep from Singing."

The song doesn't minimize life's pains, but it does encourage the listener (and the singer) to keep on embracing the joys of life and music.

> *Through all the tumult and the strife*
> *I hear that music ringing.*
> *It sounds an echo in my soul.*
> *How can I keep from singing?*

Tuesday, July 12: A Balancing Act

We are attempting to alternate between activity and rest here in the Weisblat household. I think we've ALMOST got the pattern down.

This past weekend we aimed for no more than one major event per day. This practice involved trade-offs: we went to a concert instead of the town garden tour, for example. In general, it worked, however.

Friday's big activity was probably the highlight of Taffy's weekend. We cruised the car up the highway to have lunch at the Putney Inn with her brother Bruce, who lives in Vermont.

As we crossed the border into Vermont, a state in which she spent every summer as a child, Taffy informed me that it looked and smelled much better than Massachusetts.

There are some quirks of character that dementia has trouble changing. All my life she has told me this. And all my life I have failed to perceive much difference between the trees and hills on either side of the state line.

When we arrived in Putney both siblings looked happy. Taffy spent much of lunch gazing at her brother and repeating that she loved him.

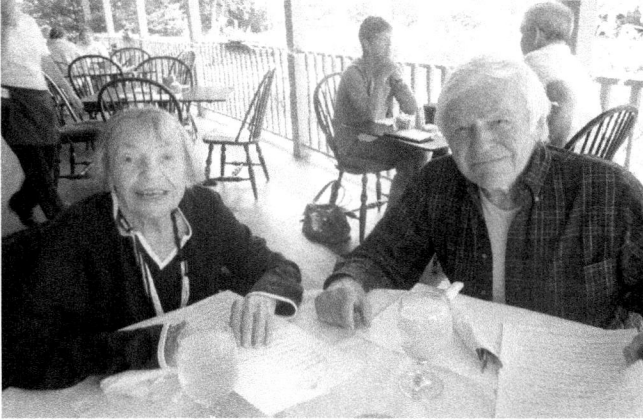

As she gazed I managed to have a nice conversation with my uncle. He turned 90 in June and seemed very fit and fun. He has always looked up to his big sister and continues to care about her deeply. He is also very sweet and dear to me.

Saturday's highlight was this week's Mohawk Trail Concert. Taffy waxed slightly critical (luckily not too loudly) of soprano Lucy Shelton, the star of the first half of the program. I guess when you have dementia making out lyrics in English is difficult enough. Hearing someone sing in German, French, and Polish(!) leaves you a bit cold.

My mother positively purred throughout the second half, however, which featured Schubert's Trout Quintet. As an added bonus a man brought his wife's service dog over during intermission to say hello to Taffy. She tried to get them to sit with her but forgave the man for returning to his wife when he gave her a kiss.

An additional treat on Saturday came in the form of a very brief visit from our once-and-future neighbors Ken and Peter. They drove up from New York to check on the progress of their house being built around the corner and stopped in long enough to say hello and to allow their dogs a chance to re-bond with our own Truffle.

After staying up late on Saturday Taffy slept in on Sunday but was wide awake for cocktails with our neighbors the Purdys in the late afternoon. Peter Purdy didn't seem to mind her asking repeatedly why his shirt said "World's Best Grandpa," although he may avoid the shirt next time we visit.

Each day we spent at least a little time by the water. Taffy still hasn't made it in for a swim (mountain-stream water is really very, VERY cold), but she loves to sit in the shade and gaze at the water and the trees.

The dog and I had lovely swims. Truffle gladly let me take off her current fashion accessory, the Cone of Shame, so that she could get into the water.

Unfortunately, our dear dog, the only member of the household aside from me who is supposed to be in perfect health, has spent a lot of time (translation: we have spent a lot of money) at the vet lately. After many expensive tests we have learned that she has a nasty infection on and in her feet. She now wears the Cone to keep her from biting those feet as they heal.

Taffy tries to remove the Cone about 15 times per day. Sadly for her but happily for Truffle's general well-being, my mother can no longer unfasten Truffle's collar.

All in all, I think our weekend was a huge success—a nice balance of company, sunshine, and rest.

The weekend did reveal one new quirk Taffy has developed that may require some diplomacy on my part. During our visit with her brother—and again with Peter and Ken and the Purdys—I was quite firmly instructed not to talk.

Have I mentioned before that my mother has lost her tact? To tell you the truth, tact was never her strong suit. Now it's a suit that doesn't appear at all in the hand of cards fate has dealt her.

Luckily, sensitivity isn't MY strong suit so I can laugh off being told to shut up. And to tell you the truth again it takes more than a command from a determined mother to stem the flow of my conversation.

Nevertheless, I can see a new balancing act looming in the near future: allowing her enough time to shine in company without feeling stepped on myself.

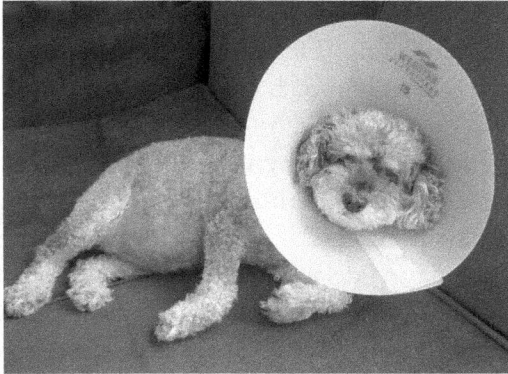

Tuesday, July 19: A Breath of Fresh Air

Living with my mother in her current state of health often focuses my brain on truths I ought to know but have managed to miss—even when they have been right in front of me for years.

One of these is the health-giving nature of fresh air. Scientists theorize about the physiological and psychological effects of the negative ions in fresh air. I wouldn't know a negative ion from a positive one if I could see it, but I can certainly observe its effects at the macro level.

Recently as we sat by the water gazing at the greenery and the blue sky Taffy made one of what one of her fans calls her "Pooh" pronouncements.

"I am breathing in and out," she said. "In and out. It makes me feel good."

It suddenly hit me that one of the reasons she is thriving since returning to our country home in Massachusetts is the abundance of fresh air.

During the last month or so of our sojourn in Virginia we ran the air conditioning in our apartment frequently.

I opened windows whenever I could. The apartment isn't designed to circulate fresh air very well, however. It has relatively small windows on only one side of each room.

When it got hot and humid outside, my mother wilted inside the apartment. And she got pretty warm when I tried to take her out as well. So the air conditioning was a boon.

Here in Massachusetts we have the luxury of not needing or wanting air conditioning. On all but the very hottest nights (of which we have only a few each year) a breeze makes its way into the bedrooms.

And in the summer (and even the fall!) we try to spend time by the water on every sunny afternoon.

Sometimes swimming isn't possible for my mother, who so far has decided each day to delay making her way into the chilly Dam until the next day. Nevertheless, just being near the water gives us the feeling of being a little cooler and a little more serene.

Like music, fresh air makes my mother bloom noticeably.

The fresh air of Massachusetts has its limits. In the winter, the dog and I still manage to garner its benefits by sauntering down the road in the snow.

My mother's snow-sauntering days are past, however, and the mere thought of opening a window during a New England winter causes her to shiver dramatically. At that time of year Virginia can provide more fresh air and more sunshine. For now, we are soaking them up in Massachusetts.

Not every day is a perky day for my mother. Yesterday clouds dimmed the blue skies, and Taffy was tired from a busy weekend. Nevertheless, by and large we count ourselves lucky to breathe the air of home. In and out, in and out.

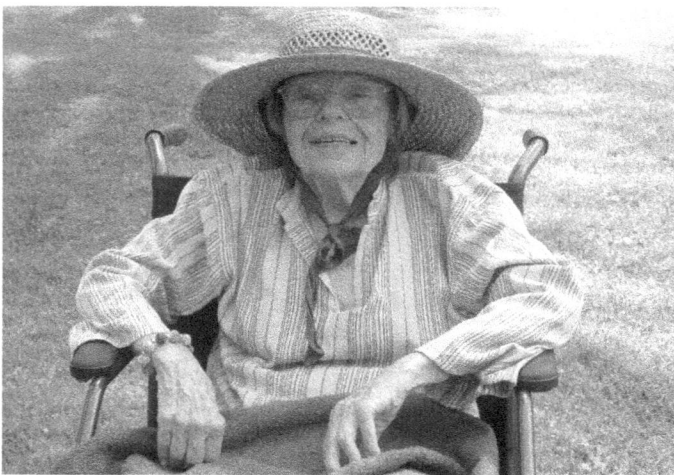

Friday, July 22: Still Listening

Last weekend Taffy and I attended Mohawk Trail Concerts' annual Bolcom and Morris offering.

Composer/pianist William Bolcom and mezzo-soprano Joan Morris are special favorites of MTC audiences and of the Weisblats as well. As they always do, the husband and wife anchored the evening with their "Songs from Theater, Film, and Cabaret."

Taffy adored the selections, which ranged from a 1909 tune to recent works. She sang along lustily on "I've Got Rings on My Fingers" and sighed appropriately as Joan expressively acted out "Can't We Be Friends?"

In between the Bolcoms' duets two pianists performed works by Bill Bolcom. Estela Olevsky, a Mohawk Trail Concerts regular who always demonstrates passion and precision, breezed through the challenging, complex "Estela: Rag Latino," named after her.

The versatile Lucas Wong played several of Bill's short works for piano … from memory. (He made this look easy, but I know it couldn't have been.) These included rags, a piano transcription of an aria from the Bolcom opera *A View from the Bridge*, and several "Bagatelles."

One of the bagatelles brought tears to my eyes. Wong described this composition as a musical illustration of the process of memory loss. A minor piece called "valse oubliable" (forgettable waltz), it moved in fits and starts and eventually just trailed away.

As the ending faded off, Taffy still appeared to be listening to something. I'm not sure she understood what the music was supposed to be about, but it certainly spoke to her.

I may be growing fanciful, but it seems to me that the mysterious moment between the last note of a piece of music—particularly this one piece of music—and the first clap of applause may well be the closest most of us can get to the sensations of dementia.

In this state my mother is suspended between past and present, emotion and intellect, knowing and not knowing. She is uncertain yet expressive, here yet not here, trailing off yet holding her place.

After the performance Joan and Bill gave both of us special hugs. I wished I had brought my camera to take a photo of them with Taffy. Maybe next year....

Tuesday, July 26: And Now for Something Completely Different....

We've had a busy week—listening to music, dining with old friends, going to church, and experiencing a reunion with my mother's two siblings.

Lura (83) was driven north by her daughter Jennifer. Bruce (90) drove himself south, bless his heart. Both looked great. And both were happy to share BLTs and their mother's chocolate cake with their sister.

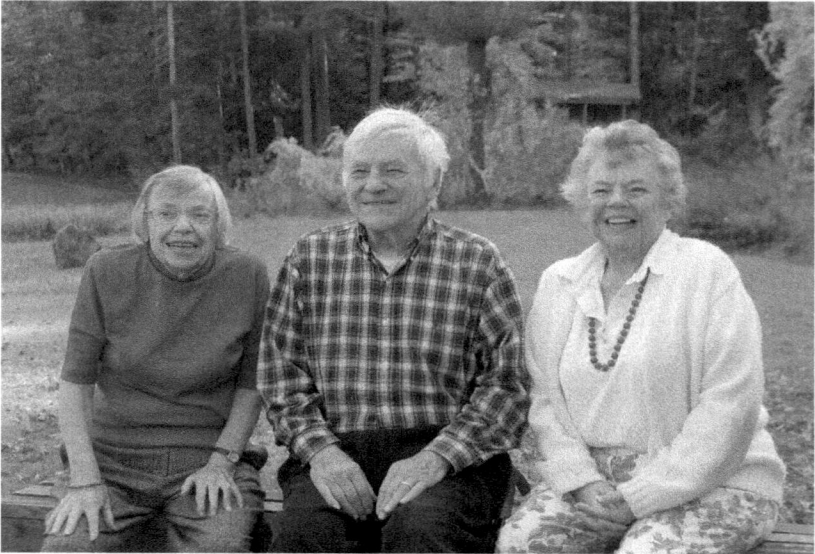

Taffy (left) with Bruce and Lura in 2008

If seeing her sister and brother was the high point of Taffy's week, the heat we have been experiencing was probably the low point. She made it through the steamy weather, however, mostly by spending a lot of time sitting quietly by the water.

I'm not a poet, but watching my mother gaze at clouds one hot afternoon inspired me to write a sort-of poem. (I promise not to be inspired too often.)

Heat Wave

An old woman watches clouds drift by.
She watched them as a child
But couldn't find the time as an adult.
Today in renewed childhood she looks skyward once more,
Relishing the fluffy patterns
In the heavens and in her imagination.
She moves so little that her body mimics death
Yet her concentration is full of life's force.
There by the water and the towering trees
Nothing stirs but bugs and birds,
The latter employing their wings only in isolated cooling swoops.
The flat brightness drains people and pets,
Reminding us that the sun,
Nurturing source of our intricate world,
Is a nexus of unstoppable waves,
Of impersonal energy that can blind and burn.
All of life—especially end of life—is a web of duality,
A negotiation with death.
Yet sitting motionless in the shade of an afternoon …
Chatting with friends,
Tracing the clouds,
And watching the water shimmer ever so slightly
As it reflects the greens, blues, and whites around us …
We cultivate the illusion that the moment can last forever.
Time is suspended. Heat is suspended. Death is suspended.
We know it's an illusion.
We embrace it nonetheless.

July Meditation: Helping Hands

Most of the pages of this book are vignettes, backstory about Taffy, or rambling thoughts about our overall situation. This essay differs in being just plain descriptive. A friend said that it would be helpful if I explained how much help we had for Taffy and how we found these people.

As I hope you can tell from reading these pages, I didn't take care of Taffy all by myself. We were lucky enough to live in a vibrant community of caring people. We were also lucky enough (that is, Taffy was!) to be able to afford to hire people to help with her.

Dementia offers many surprises to those who have it and to their families. One of the biggest ones, as far as I am concerned, is the sudden realization that even the most excellent standard health insurance doesn't cover care for people who need help because they are suffering from dementia. Long-term-care policies often do cover this help, but by the time Taffy thought about applying for such a policy she was ineligible. Needless to say, I am hoping to take out long-term-care insurance for myself ... as soon as I can afford it!

Meanwhile, as I said, luckily Taffy had a pension and some savings in addition to her social security. So she had help for the last year and a half of her life. With me in the house to cover nights and odd hours, hiring help was still less expensive than a nursing home would have been. And it was much more comfortable for Taffy.

We began hiring people gradually. We consulted Joan Miller Sutton when we arrived in Virginia to begin exploring living near my brother David's family. David had a friend whose parents had been working with Joan for a couple of years so she came highly recommended.

Joan is a vivacious woman who runs a business called Connections for Seniors. Under this rubric she has two main jobs. One is to spend an hour or two every week or so with senior clients suffering from dementia. Sometimes she visits with them at home; sometimes she takes them out for a drive or a snack. Joan draws her clients out in conversation, asking questions (but not worrying whether the answers make a lot of sense) and eliciting any memories she can. She also tends to stimulate their senses by wearing bright clothing and engaging them in simple reading and motor activities.

When Joan met Taffy, they clicked instantly. (I have a feeling Joan clicks with all of her clients!) Joan's gentle conversation made Taffy laugh and brought forth memories I didn't know my mother still had in her head. Although Taffy had at one time been completely fluent in French, in recent years she had no longer been able to speak or understand much of the language. Somehow or other, however, when Joan said, "Tell me something in French," a complete French sentence would pop out of Taffy's mouth.

Joan also helps family members of her clients figure out how best to keep those clients happy. And she is a one-stop resource for elder care in Northern Virginia. After her first meeting with Taffy she emailed my brother and me a general assessment of Taffy's dementia, along with suggestions for suitable physical therapists, primary-care physicians, home-care agencies, and adult day-care centers. Although she knew we weren't necessarily ready to place Taffy in an extended-care facility, she gave us the names of a couple of nearby places to visit (describing the advantages and disadvantages of each) so we could have an idea of what was offered just in case we decided to take that route at some point. Joan was a gold mine, and without her we would have been scrambling a lot more than we did.

She suggested that we employ either home health aides or adult day care to stimulate Taffy and give me a break from care. Taffy was already dealing with a new environment, having just moved to Virginia, so we chose to minimize disruption by hiring an aide to come in for a few days a week rather than try day care. We went through an agency Joan recommended. Synergy Home Care worked very hard to find a pleasant, intelligent companion for Taffy. The one who came most often was named Pertina Wallace. She stayed with us for six months, until we went home to Massachusetts for the summer.

Agencies have advantages and disadvantages relative to individual aides. Agencies are more expensive than most privately found aides, but the agency does all the vetting for the family. It also takes care of all the relevant taxes and unemployment payments. In general, Pertina was a great fit for us. Her only flaw—and this was the agency's policy, not something that originated with Pertina—was that she was a little too respectful to Taffy. She called her "Mrs. Weisblat" and was quite restrained with her.

Unfortunately, by the time we met Pertina Taffy barely remembered that her last name was Weisblat (she had pretty much forgotten her marriage). And she had regressed enough into childhood that she was more interested in being hugged than in being respected. Nevertheless, we could not have done without Pertina and the agency.

As we prepared to return to Massachusetts, I began calling around to find an aide or aides near our home in Hawley. I knew that there were no agencies nearby. I was lucky, however, to be looking for help in a small community in which everyone knew everyone else.

I put out the word that I was looking and visited a couple of bulletin boards online. When I learned that a licensed certified nursing assistant and home health aide named Pam Gerry who lived 15 minutes from our home had recently lost a patient and was looking for work, it was easy to find someone who knew her; our minister spoke highly of her. I called Pam, and her cheerful voice on the phone made me realize that I had found someone who would relate to Taffy.

The minute they met, it was clear that Pam was an ideal friend and caregiver for Taffy. They played games. They went on outings. They talked to the dog and cat by the hour. Pam was great at anticipating what medicines, toys, and equipment Taffy might need. At her suggestion, for example, we replaced the unpopular oral thermometer with one we could pop in and out of Taffy's ear. We also purchased a long pillow that supported our patient's back in bed. I was grateful for Pam's ideas and feedback.

Pam began by coming two to three days a week for a few hours. As Taffy grew weaker, we increased both the days and the hours. When we found that we needed help six and then seven days a week, Pam recommended people with whom she had worked in the past to supplement her help.

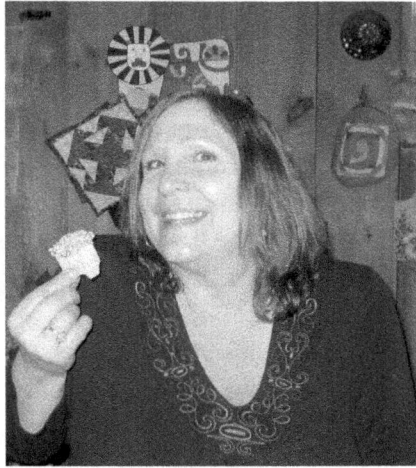

*Our wonderful Pam
samples her dip
(see recipe at end of chapter).*

As luck would have it, we had already met both of them. In fact, one of them, Jennifer Rich, was a neighbor whom we had known for decades. (We were aware that she was a home-health aide; we just hadn't realized she was looking for additional work.)

Jen was a lifeline for us since she lived only five minutes from our house. Eventually, we reached the point at which I became nervous about putting Taffy to bed by myself. Lifting her to change her into her pajamas stymied me. Although she weighed very little, her tiny body was dead weight in the evenings when she was tired. I became spooked when I almost dropped her one evening. Jen said she would come by in the evenings when she could to give me a hand.

Like Pam, Jen was adored by Taffy. The best caregivers seem to connect on an almost subconscious level with the people they tend. Taffy always greeted Jen's "Hello, Beautiful" with a huge smile.

Our other caregiver, Joan De Gusto, came to help out in the evenings during which Jen wasn't free. Joan is a fey soul who designs reproduction vintage clothing in addition to working as an aide and loves to sing. Taffy had fun playing with whatever Joan was wearing, and they spent the half hour or so before bedtime listening to music and looking at books and magazines. Like Pam and Jen, Joan provided care that combined love and whimsy and soothed both my mother and me.

In the last few months of her life, as you will see later in this book, Taffy was placed under hospice care by a physician. A hospice aide (usually the competent, smiling Jackie Baker) came to help her get dressed in the morning, first a few days a week and eventually daily. Taffy usually needed to take a nap right after getting dressed and eating breakfast so with this system we could have Pam or Jen come later in the day when she was waking up from her nap, giving me more coverage and giving Taffy more quality time.

Hospice is an odd yet wonderful organization. It appears to vary by state. When I started to look into it before we left Virginia, it appeared that Taffy would have qualified for hospice care in that state even then because she could not get around without help and had a low body-mass index. In Massachusetts, however, we had to wait until the doctors really thought she had less than six months to live, body-mass index or no body-mass index.

I didn't always agree with the hospice nurses and social workers when it came to Taffy's care. Their mission is to let an illness take its course, almost to welcome death. Taffy and I were defiant of death almost to the end. Nevertheless, they respected my views even when they couldn't agree with me. And they provided not only an aide every morning but nurses and social workers to talk to whenever we needed them—even late at night. Despite all the help we had, I was often alone with Taffy physically. I knew, however, that I was never completely alone with her spiritually. And that was a huge relief.

Taffy also had an assigned hospice volunteer, a darling great-grandmother named Rose Kiablick. Rose loved to come chat every week and often brought Taffy homemade treats. Toward the end, when Taffy was napping more and more, Rose just put her arm around Taffy and held her hand. Sadly, Rose died suddenly not long after Taffy. I grieved for the family whom she obviously adored.

All in all, I am enormously grateful for the care Taffy and her family received over the last year or so of her life. As I have indicated, part of the care we received was a matter of luck.

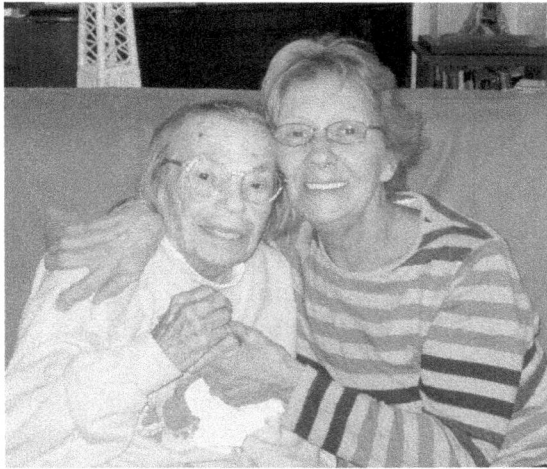

Taffy with Rose

Part of the source of the excellence of Taffy's care stemmed from my mother's cheerful nature. Except when she was having one of her contrary, infection-driven days, she was fun to be with. All her caregivers responded to that sense of fun.

I think it also helped that I treated all of the people who helped us not as employees but as partners, as the experts they were in caring for people in Taffy's condition. Respect and good humor make life easier for everyone in these situations. Occasionally, our aides would do a little housework when Taffy was sleeping; Pam in particular hated to be idle so she was quick to pick up a broom or fold laundry. (I HATE folding laundry and probably as a consequence do it very poorly.) I didn't expect them to do housework, however. They had their hands full taking care of Taffy.

I hug the hospice workers when I see them, and I have sweet memories of all of our helpers. Joan Sutton, Pam, and Jen in particular have become friends with whom I am still in touch. In fact, I see Pam on a regular basis when she comes to help me organize myself and my business. It's a task that I fear will never end. Luckily, we're having such a good time working together that we don't want it to end. From time to time we see a photo of Taffy or find ourselves doing something that she liked to do, and we smile at each other.

July Recipe: Pam's Traveling Spinach and Artichoke Dip

This recipe comes from our wonderful Pam Gerry. She says it has traveled up and down the east coast of the United States, and I can see why. Taffy loved its vegetably cheesiness.

Ingredients:

1 small onion, finely chopped
6 large cloves garlic, minced
a tiny bit of extra-virgin olive oil (and/or butter) as needed for frying
1 10-ounce package frozen spinach, thawed and squeezed to get the water out
1 14-ounce can artichoke hearts, drained
1 cup grated Parmesan and/or Romano cheese, plus 4 tablespoons later
2 tablespoons lemon juice
1/2 cup mayonnaise
1 8-ounce brick cream cheese (light cream cheese is fine), softened
1/4 cup bread crumbs (I used panko crumbs.)

Instructions:

Preheat the oven to 375 degrees.

In a small frying pan sauté the onion and garlic pieces in the oil and/or butter until the vegetables soften.

In a food processor combine the spinach and the artichoke hearts. Pulse to make them very small. Add the cup of cheese, the lemon juice, the mayonnaise, the cream cheese, and the sautéed vegetables. Pulse again to combine thoroughly.

If you don't have a food processor, chop the artichoke hearts well before beating them together with the rest of the ingredients.

Place the mixture in a 2-quart baking dish. Sprinkle the top with the bread crumbs and remaining cheese.

Bake until the dip is brown around the edges, about 20 minutes. Serve with chips, sliced vegetables, or bread.

Makes about 4 cups.

AUGUST
A Month of Crises

Tuesday, August 2: Gender Identity

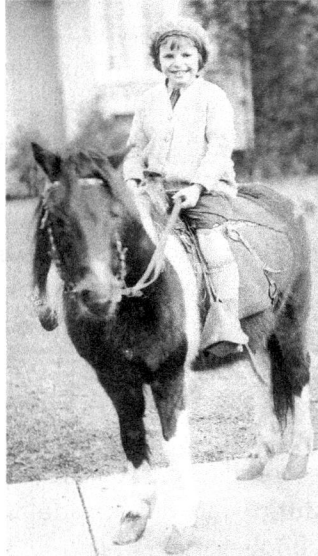

I have written before in these pages about my mother's apparent regression to childhood. We think she is somewhere between three and four years old at this point.

Today's topic is a new realm in which she has started mimicking very young children. She is becoming concerned about her gender.

Most of the time she is fairly certain she is a girl. She mentions this in particular when she is dressing or undressing and therefore exposing "girl" parts. "I'm a girl," she informs me as I help her put on her pajamas. "Did you know that?" Her tone is just a little surprised.

I assure her that I do know and that she has always been a girl as far as I know. Just for good measure I mention that the cat, the dog, and I are girls as well.

The other evening she elaborated a bit on this theme as we chatted with our friend Peter.

"I'm not sure whether I'm a girl or a boy," she said.

We replied that we were pretty sure she was a girl.

"For a long time I didn't know what I was," she noted. "I thought maybe I was a boy. Then when I got to be about eleven and I got ... things [here she cupped her breasts] ... I decided I was a girl."

The very young Taffy was indeed rather boyish. She was a definite tomboy. Her hairstyle, then as now, was a Dutch boy bob, and she was frequently told she looked like Jackie Coogan, a child star who appeared in many popular films including *The Kid* (1921). (Yes, he grew up to be Uncle Fester on *The Addams Family!*)

Taffy resisted her horrified grandmother's attempts to feminize her—and she detested most dolls. Being a girly girl myself I have always been sad that her curly-haired sister Lura got the collectible dolls in the family, including Shirley Temple and Scarlett O'Hara.

Taffy always said she beat up her little brother frequently ... until he became bigger and stronger than she. At that point she wisely stopped picking fights.

As an adult she was never super feminine, although she certainly cultivated the art of flirtation. I never got an exact count on the number of fiancés she had, but they were numerous. She didn't like to hurt boys' feelings when they cared enough to ask her to marry them, she explained to me once.

She always assured my brother and me that our father was the only one from whom she took a ring—although she did manage to order sterling flatware wholesale from the previous fiancé's uncle, who was a jeweler. (She cleverly had her maiden initial inscribed rather than the fiancé's.)

Today she is a bit more feminine in appearance than she was during most of her adult life, when she favored tailored clothing. I choose her clothes every day and tend to like pink ... and hats. (Did I mention that I am a doll-loving girly girl?)

Despite Taffy's feminine appearance gender comes up more and more frequently in her conversation.

Perhaps at some point she will become too young again in her head to notice it. In a way this ultimate deconstruction of gender might be fascinating; living in a pre-gendered body (or post-gendered body), Taffy would to some extent be a cultural critic's dream.

What would it be like to be so far outside of social conditioning that gender had no meaning? That's the sort of question psychologists, sociologists, and historians love to ask. On the other hand, if she gets to that point Taffy won't be able to tell us what it is like because she will be incapable of analysis.

For now, gender is something she seems to need to establish anew as she needs to establish so much—who people are, where rooms in the house are, what day it is, where home is.

Wednesday, August 10: Hearts and Raisins

Taffy is currently in the hospital. I'll fill you in on that story soon, but meanwhile here is an essay I drafted but wasn't able to finish yesterday just before we took her to the emergency room. I am polishing it in her hospital room.

The essay ruminates on the brain and the heart.

Blaise Pascal famously wrote, "Le cœur a ses raisons, que la raison ne connaît point." ("The heart has reasons of which reason knows nothing.")

I believe it was P.G. Wodehouse who had a character say, "The heart has raisins of which raisins know nothing." The statement is a very silly parody, but one that has always tickled my funny bone—and my mother's.

I am frequently reminded of the truth of Pascal's thought when I deal with my mother. Her brain and reasoning power aren't always there. There's a lot more to a person than her brain, however, as she showed again last week.

On Friday Taffy had a minor surgical procedure, an upper endoscopy. Her doctor had suggested that putting a scope down her esophagus and widening (dilating) it would make it easier for her to swallow and therefore easier for her to eat a bit more. She has a large hiatal hernia that has been pushing in on the esophagus and narrowing it.

Although the procedure took longer than expected—EVERYTHING takes longer than expected when one is almost 93—it seemed to go pretty well.

It helped that the operating doctor was from India and the nurse was Cinni Donovan, who with her husband Ivy grows wonderful organic potatoes at Donovan Farm here in Hawley, Massachusetts. That combination of places she loves seemed ideal for Taffy.

Despite this winning combination, waking Taffy up after the operation proved almost as rocky as Hawley's hills.

At first Cinni said it would only be a few minutes and had me stay in the waiting room.

Eventually, however, she came to get me since Taffy was proving unresponsive.

I held Taffy's hand and suggested she wake up. Almost immediately I felt a little squeeze back on my hand—actually a big squeeze. (Did I mention that last time Taffy had a little procedure she bent my left thumb back so much that it still hurts when I try to use it?)

"She knows your voice," said Cinni. "That's great."

She suggested I stay with Taffy as she woke up and keep talking. It took a while, but eventually we had the patient up and moving. She came home cheerfully if a little sleepily and does seem to be eating slightly better than before the endoscopy.

On the average day, Taffy asks who I am a lot. Sometimes she remembers my name; more often she has no idea what it is. She has only the vaguest idea of our relationship; she occasionally refers to me as her daughter but is more likely to call me her sister, her friend, or just plain "her."

I don't let this bother me because there isn't much I can do about it. I figure it's my job to love her the way she is now rather than to pursue the thankless task of trying to make her revert to the way she used to be.

Nevertheless, it was gratifying to learn the other day that my voice struck a chord when my mother was in need.

Taffy's brain may be a little iffy, but her heart is full of raisins.

Wednesday, August 17: Dodging a Bullet

We've been on a wild roller coaster this week in the Weisblat household. Fortunately, the ride is over—at least for the moment. My mother is home surrounded by family and friends. She's a little tired, of course, but then so are the rest of us!

It started, as my previous entry indicated, last Tuesday. Taffy had been experiencing ups and downs—including a bout or two of fever—for a couple of days.

Nevertheless, it wasn't until she awoke on Tuesday with a completely new symptom, shaking, that her caregiver Pam and I decided it was time to call the doctor. The doctor referred us to the emergency room of the hospital in our county seat of Greenfield, Massachusetts. Off we went.

As she often does in public, Taffy perked up in the E.R. (I perked up, too, since the two doctors we saw were extremely attractive and personable young men.) She enjoyed chatting with the staff and was pleased when the X-Ray technician opined that Taffy was wearing the "cutest socks ever."

As the day turned into evening and the evening turned into night, however, she became tired. Around 9:30 p.m. we were told that her problem had been identified. She had a little hole in her stomach that was leaking all sorts of things out into the rest of her body. To make matters worse, that stomach hole was in her chest, thanks to her hiatal hernia.

The doctors talked me through our options, and I relayed them to my brother in Virginia by phone.

One option was surgery. This would have to be done at the Greenfield facility's sister hospital in Springfield (just over a half hour farther from home) since the Springfield hospital had better chest surgeons.

If we were going to move her to Springfield, the cute doctors told us, we should do it right away. The faster we addressed the problem, the easier it would be to solve. And if she went septic during the night in Greenfield, it would be nearly impossible to get her down to Springfield for surgery.

The other option was leaving the thing alone and waiting to see whether it healed itself. The doctors didn't present this as a very strong option, but they did present it, particularly since they knew we might not want to pursue surgery on our 92-year-old mother.

Taffy, bless her, didn't understand what was going on at all but told me that she would do whatever her family wanted.

Frankly, my brother and I felt that we needed more information. We agreed to have Taffy moved to Springfield so we could consult with the surgeons there.

Taffy and I arrived in Springfield by ambulance between one and two in the morning, and tests continued throughout the night. At eight in the morning the surgeon who was considering operating asked me for a decision. I asked her what she would do if her own mother were in this situation.

She informed me that, although Taffy had a 75-percent chance of living through the surgery, its aftermath would entail months of rehabilitation in a strange facility with tubes in and out of her body. My brother and I quickly decided that our mother's frailty in general and her dementia in particular rendered that option inconceivable.

The surgeons in Springfield then tried a procedure in which they attempted to place a tube through Taffy's nose down her esophagus. They said this would increase the chances that her stomach hole might heal. Unfortunately, the procedure terrified her, and she resisted so much that they couldn't succeed.

A very nice young surgeon told me that it would be possible to try this procedure after sedating Taffy—but added that the sedation could be dangerous at her age and that she would very likely pull out the tube once she woke up. We abandoned the idea.

I asked the doctors to transfer Taffy back to the hospital in Greenfield at this point. It didn't sound as though her chances of survival were huge, and I wanted to have her closer to home where it would be easier for my brother David's family and me to go back and forth from our house to the hospital (kind neighbors were caring for our pets, but we couldn't ask them to do this forever)—and where friends could come visit her.

David arrived by plane just before the ambulance took Taffy back to Greenfield Wednesday afternoon. His wife Leigh and son Michael drove into our yard in Hawley late that night.

The doctor in Greenfield informed us that the nurses would observe Taffy for a couple of additional days, pumping antibiotics and liquids into her system but feeding her nothing. If the hole showed any signs of healing after that, they would continue. If not, they would send her home with hospice care.

Thursday was a discouraging day since our little mother was completely exhausted and had no fuel going into her body. I must admit to getting a bit tearful from time to time, although I was careful not to cry outright in front of Taffy.

Thursday afternoon the nurses added a little glucose to the fluids in the I.V. Taffy perked up slightly and demanded to go home and to eat food. She wanted ice cream in particular.

It was hard to tell her that we couldn't give it to her for the moment ... and harder still to admit to ourselves that she might never be able to enjoy ice cream again.

Friday morning the doctors tested Taffy's stomach again. They said they wouldn't know for some time what the results were. So the rest of the family went home to rest and swim while our dear caregiver Pam kept Taffy company in the hospital.

When we got home to change into our swimsuits we found a telephone message from Pam. She said that the doctor hadn't shared the test results with her but added that she was hopeful. Taffy had been allowed a liquid snack.

Our minister Cara, who was visiting the hospital at the time, wrote me an email about this moment. "I was actually there," she told me, "when the nurse suddenly brought in a tiny cup of apple juice and a tiny cup of strawberry jello (pink!)... I wish you could have seen Jan relish those two things! It was wonderful fun!"

I called the hospital. The doctor informed me that our mother was indeed healing on her own. Some people are just hard to kill.

She came home on Sunday with the help of hospice. Sandra, the hospice nurse on duty over the weekend, wasn't sure that Taffy was actually a candidate for hospice services despite the doctor's recommendation that hospice become involved.

"I went for a walk down the hall with your mother in her cute little sneakers," she told me. "She was adorable. I didn't see a woman in decline. I saw a woman with a strong will to live."

Nevertheless, she approved Taffy for hospice services—which included a very convenient hospital bed for her to use on her return home—pending a future review. "After all," Sandra informed me, "there are worse things than being dropped by hospice."

There are indeed.

Taffy is much weaker after her recent hospital adventures. Nevertheless, she is beginning to eat a bit and regain some strength. She has enjoyed having her whole family around, and she and our dog Truffle had a joyful reunion when she returned from the hospital.

She has begun to venture back outdoors into the sunshine. And she has had lots of chats with people she loves, including our friend Anna from Boston, who brought her new puppy Louis to visit Taffy for a little pet therapy.

Taffy is even beginning to help around the house again. Last night she mixed ingredients for dinner.

I don't delude myself that my mother will last forever. The past week has shown all of us how frail she is and how much her dementia will affect any health decisions we make about her in the future.

Nevertheless, I am happy to have her with us a little longer. The little girl she has become grows sweeter and sweeter each day, and life seems more and more precious to her as she holds people's hands, gazes at the trees about us, and giggles at silly jokes.

We'll try to savor each small adventure as the days and months go by. And we'll celebrate dodging last week's bullet.

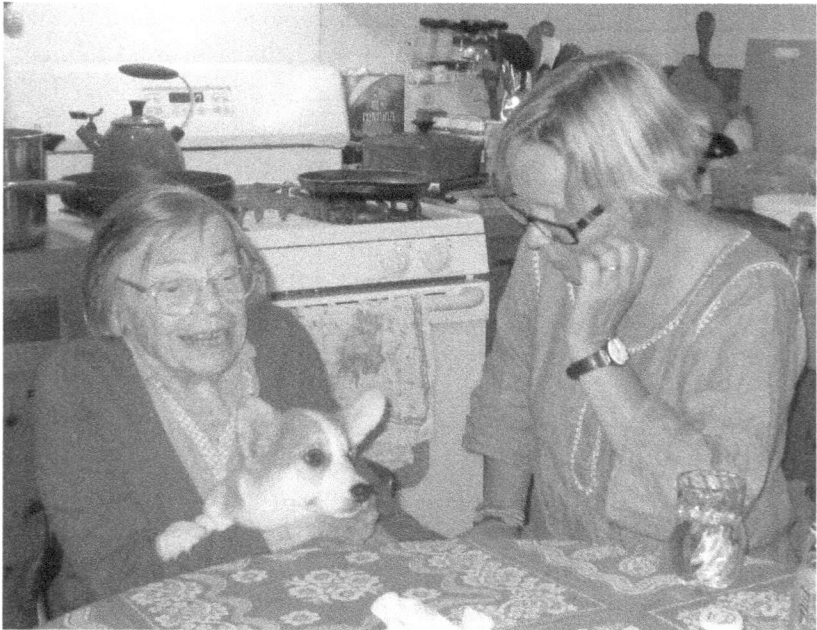

Home with Anna and Louis

Wednesday, August 24: Shaken but Smiling

Yesterday's east-coast earthquake made no noticeable dents in Hawley, Massachusetts.

I felt a bit shaken nonetheless by the end of the day. It was not a day I would care to repeat. I am hugely grateful for the many blessings I enjoyed and continue to enjoy, however.

I knew something was a little off with my mother when she started getting up at five that morning. Lately she had been catching up on the rest she lost while in the hospital two weeks ago so she had been sleeping late, a habit of which I heartily approved.

I tried to get her to go back to sleep yesterday morning, but her little body popped out of bed so many times that eventually I bowed to fate and let her get up.

As the day went by she appeared weaker and weaker. By late afternoon, she could hardly stand with help. Her speech made less and less sense—although she was still eager to make conversation, holding my hand or Pam's as she talked and looking into our eyes as she rambled.

She was also hallucinating to some extent, seeing people and things in the room we simply could not see. At night she saw her mother, a vision with symbolism it is hard to miss.

But ... as they say on television ... that's not all. We now have another patient in the Weisblat family!

Our generous neighbor Alice offered in the afternoon to pick up our farm share at Wilder Brook Farm since it was clear that my mother wasn't really capable of going there in the car. We accepted gratefully.

At about 5:30 Alice drove into the driveway and came in with all sorts of lovely things—beans, tomatoes, beets, greens, tender carrots, garlic, and simply spectacular flowers. As Alice started to back out of the driveway we heard a high-pitched, frightened (and frightening) squeal.

I ran out the door and called the dog. After a moment Truffle shakily emerged from behind Alice's rear wheel, where she had apparently been resting unbeknownst to either Alice or me. Truffle was having a lot of trouble maneuvering the rear portion of her body so I carried her inside, and Alice helped me settle her on a quilt on the floor.

Alas, Truffle's doctor was gone for the day. So was the cat's (who has been known to take care of Truffle in a pinch). Their answering services referred me to the pet emergency hospital in South Deerfield, about 45 minutes away.

Alice offered to stay with my mother while I took Truffle to the hospital, but since my mother was in such bad shape—and since I knew Alice would have trouble lifting her if she fell—I didn't feel that I could accept her offer, although I certainly treasured it.

I called Pam, who (bless her heart!) said she would leave her almost cooked dinner and her very understanding husband to come help out. She finished feeding Taffy and settled her down for the night while Truffle and I sped in the car to South Deerfield.

We have yet to determine what precisely is going on with my mother, who is even weaker and vaguer today. Is she dying quickly? Is she suffering from a recurrence of the hole in her stomach? Is this a new stage of her dementia?

The hospice nurse says that Taffy MAY be dying but that she may also be just a little weak and in need of even more rest. She is certainly sleeping today away. Time will tell.

As for Truffle, she will definitely return home—but not until after surgery, which will probably take place tomorrow.

As an aside, here's a true story about Truffle. When the vet called this morning to update me on the pooch's status, I asked, "How IS Truffle?"

"Truffle is adorable," she replied.

"I knew that," I said. I went on to ask about Truffle's actual state of health, although it was nice to know that even with an I.V. hooked up to her paw my dog hadn't lost her charm.

As I noted earlier, I certainly don't want to repeat yesterday's stress anytime soon. And yet I still find things to be grateful for.

One is exercise. I'm not technically what anyone would call physically fit. Nevertheless, I try each day to do something that moves and stretches my body. At the moment my exercise of choice is swimming; it will change to walking as soon as the weather gets much colder. I am lucky enough to be able to swim in a simply gorgeous setting. As soon as I get into the water—well, as soon as I get used to the water, which is extremely cold—any anxiety or stress I have been feeling gets washed away. Yesterday my mother was still well enough to sit by the water's edge and watch me glide along.

My friends and relatives are another blessing. My neighbor Alice is not the only person who has helped over the last few weeks, although she is the closest to hand (and one who never minds a call, even when she's working). Betsy and Jack visit my mother and cheerfully perform labor—hanging quilts, moving beds, folding inflatable kayaks. Erwin and Linda, who raise lambs, have brought tiny lamb chops to tempt Taffy's palate. Esther has offered to run errands. Susan stops by with flowers and zucchini brownies. Cara comes just to talk to Taffy. Cynthia, Russ, Sandy, and others are standing by to visit as needed. And the amazing Peter is planning a ramp to get Taffy in and out of the house more easily; we hope she will live to use it!

My Uncle Bruce is at the other end of the telephone line for medical and familial consultations, and many of my cousins have called and written to offer help and support. Best of all, my brother David and his family have been gentle, sweet, and loving with Taffy. David is a whiz at getting her to take her pills, demonstrating a patience I could never emulate. And then we have the wonderful Pam. Pam is the perfect aide and friend for my mother—a constant source of hugs and laughter. She can cook, too!

Finally, I am blessed that I get to sing every day—including yesterday and today. The music calms those in need around me; I sing to my mother even when she's not very responsive, and I sang to Truffle as I drove her to the puppy E.R.

Singing makes me feel wonderful. It stretches me physically (all that lung and diaphragm work) and emotionally, and it's satisfyingly creative.

I may not remember all the lyrics for my performance this coming Saturday, but I'm still glad I have one. Whatever the future may hold (I hope not too many more bad surprises!), today I feel shaken but strong. And still smiling.

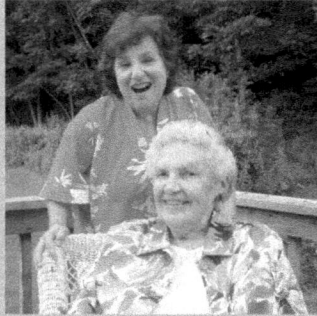

Summertime

And the Music Is Easy....

Tinky Weisblat, Soprano
Alice Parker, Piano

Saturday, August 27, at 7:30 pm
at the Green Emporium in Colrain
413-624-5122

Wednesday, August 31: Stormy Weather

The word "eventful" doesn't BEGIN to sum up the week since I last turned on my laptop and put finger to keyboard. My mother and I have made it through a couple of different kinds of stormy weather.

The first storm was a health one. Taffy's condition when I wrote last Wednesday morning was precarious. Wednesday went on to be just plain scary. My mother spent much of the day utterly unresponsive. When she opened her eyes she didn't actually look at anyone. And she didn't get out of bed. She ate and drank nothing.

Fortunately, I had both Pam and the hospice nurse, Dvora, to help me get her dressed and change her linens. (I'm not good at either task when she's lying in bed.)

Dvora predicted that we would know more about my mother's status—for better or for worse—within a day or two.

I actually knew more about it (for better!) that evening.

At about 5:30 I decided to practice my singing, figuring that the music might cheer her up. I peeked into her room as I was launching into the second chorus of "A Wonderful Guy."

Her hands were moving to the music.

I went to her side and was rewarded with a big smile.

By the next day Taffy was ready to get up several times, albeit in her wheelchair. By Friday she was back using her walker as though whatever it was had never happened.

I hoped she might even come to hear me sing and Alice play the piano Saturday night. On Saturday afternoon, however, she chose to accompany me to the puppy hospital to pick up the recovering Truffle, and by evening she was ready to sleep.

Pam graciously agreed to take care of both invalids (Truffle was barely moving and eating) while I zipped away to my singing engagement.

That engagement was a delight. Forecasters were busy predicting that Tropical Storm Irene was going to hit the area before midnight. Despite the threat of inclement weather, a large crowd of music lovers, food lovers, and (I admit it!) Tinky lovers gathered to hear the Divas of Hawley, Massachusetts, before the storm hit.

At the last minute Alice and I added "Stormy Weather" and "Goodnight, Irene" to our final, sing-along set. The audience and the Divas all got a kick out of singing them.

As I drove home the rain began to fall. Sunday morning the power went out … and the rain continued.

By midday on Sunday we began to hear of disasters around us. One neighbor at the bottom of the hill had water lapping at his house's edges. Another was clearing all the machinery out of his barn. A few trailers, homes, and businesses in the area had been swept away.

The Dam in which I had swum just Saturday afternoon was filled with gravel, soil, and branches. The brand-new bridge across the Dam was gone ... moving down our own Mill Brook to the Chickley River and thence to the Deerfield River, the Connecticut River, and for all I know the Atlantic Ocean.

We were cut off from the outside world since Route 8A, the road that leads away from our community, was washed out in both directions.

A kindly neighbor with a generator and a tractor brought us enough drinking and washing water to last for at least a week. He also brought ice to keep some of our cold food usable.

Other neighbors and friends brought food, stopped by with news, and organized our hill for disaster response.

On Monday morning FEMA and its state counterpart MEMA sent helicopters with personnel, expertise, and food and water to the Town Office around the corner from our house. We get very few helicopters in Hawley, and the only other people we see in fatigues are hunters. These officials were a very big deal in our very tiny town.

When neighbors first called offering to deliver some of the FEMA food I said we had plenty to eat, which was true. People were bringing by meals all the time.

I AM a food writer, however, and I couldn't resist the thought of trying an actual government-issue MRE (meal ready to eat, the stuff our armed forces get in the field). I asked them to bring one or two packages. I am particularly intrigued by the Thai Chicken! It comes with its own little heater and looks like a hoot.

By midday yesterday, miracle of miracles, our power was restored. And today, if one has an extremely sturdy car and is an extremely courageous driver, one MAY be able to get to Charlemont, the next town over. Driving Taffy's car and being a Tinky kind of driver, I'm waiting a day or two to try. I hear the National Guard(!) is helping our road crew make the road more passable.

My mother was amazing throughout the whole powerless ordeal. She did have a little trouble figuring out why it was so dark and why she couldn't get water from the tap. And she took a lot of naps.

Nevertheless, she was fairly perky when she was awake. She enjoyed having neighbors stop by to check on us. And she slept well at night. Her general aura of good health was reassuring to me since I knew it would be hard to get help for her if she needed it.

Now Taffy's body seems to know it doesn't have to be the Energizer Bunny anymore.

Yesterday she was barely awake—and she had no interest for once in going outside to sit in the fresh air. I called the hospice nurse on duty and described her symptoms—and believe it or not was told that she seems to have yet another urinary-tract infection! So she is back on antibiotics, poor dear. I hope the pills, along with Pam (who returns this morning), will help me perk Taffy up again. And I hope the probiotic yogurt I'm feeding my mother will keep the pills from causing a tropical storm in her digestive system.

Our other invalid, Truffle the dog, is still moving very slowly after her hip operation. Truffle had a low opinion of the rain on Sunday. She is obviously happy to be home resting comfortably with her family, her cat, and her toys, however.

I adore being able to bathe now that our water pump is working again—and I'm tackling the piles of laundry that stacked up while we were without power and water.

I feel for those who suffered property damage in the storm. (Happily, so far I have heard of no one who was physically hurt.) I feel fortunate that our own inconvenience was so minimal. In fact, I felt blessed for much of the duration of the storm and its aftermath.

Our friends and neighbors helped with comfort and information (Peter in New York seemed to know more about events in our area than people who were in residence!) as well as comestibles.

The local newspaper and radio station apparently made much of our town's being cut off by the storm. Ironically, it was when we were most cut off that we felt most connected. I know that feeling of connection will endure long after the roads are fixed and the bridges replaced.

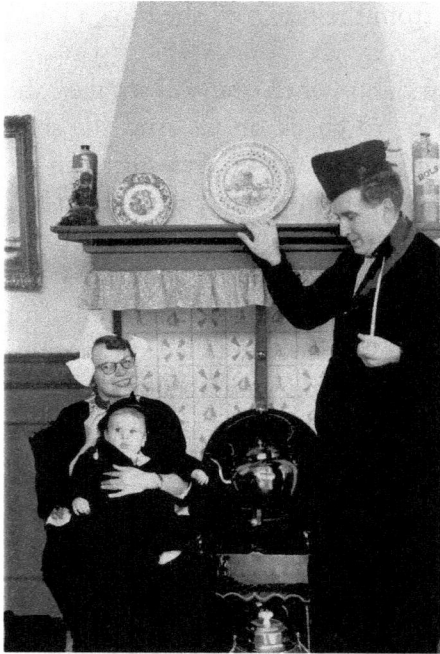

We have no photos of my family in India in 1953-1954; those were sent home to their parents and lost. This one was taken on the voyage out, in Holland.

August Meditation: A Passage to India

Americans are often most ourselves in a foreign environment—and we learn a lot about ourselves when we are immersed in other cultures.

This was particularly true of my mother. I noted in the essay on her education that her junior year abroad represented a true coming of age for Taffy/Jan. During her months in France between 1937 and 1938 she learned to be independent, learned to flirt, and gained self-confidence.

Her time in India similarly stimulated and illuminated her. She spent a total of almost four years there, but the most important year was her first, a stay with my father and my older brother (then a baby) in Bombay, now known as Mumbai, in 1953-1954. She and my father were in their mid 30s.

My father had been pondering topics for his doctoral thesis in agricultural economics. He decided that applying for a fellowship to study overseas would be a good idea. Unlike my mother he was a terrible linguist so he wanted to go to a country in which he could get by in English. India was an obvious choice. He received a Ford Foundation stipend to study the potential for non-agricultural employment in rural areas of that country. The whole family set off, ready for adventure.

Jan, Abe, and four-month-old David sailed to England in August 1953 on the first leg of their journey to India. Their ten-day trip on the S.S. America was luxurious. Friends and relatives turned out to see them off, and when they went in search of their tiny, interior stateroom they discovered that a friend of Jan's father, who was on the board of the steamship line, had mysteriously turned it into a first-class cabin. They had another happy surprise in store. Jan's travel diary reveals that her father had given the wine steward a budget to keep the couple in good spirits literally as well as figuratively.

Abe was supposed to spend a couple of months consulting with an academic adviser in England about his research. When the adviser became unavailable, the young couple spent a few weeks with old friends in England before heading on to Germany and France. Jan and little David settled into Paris, staying with a cousin of Abe who happened to live in that city, while Abe and his graduate-school pal Gene Kleinschmit toured Europe together.

Jan adored spending time in the city with which she had fallen in love as a college student. Her travel diary reveals her joy in small moments in Paris. One evening after the theater she wrote,

"I wandered into the lobby and delighted my soul further as I looked out through the colonnades at the fountains in front. I felt as tho I were re-finding Paris as I had loved it! And the life—the magnetic life of the city as I saw it again wandering through the streets, the narrow streets thronged with shops and people."

As always she adored French food. Her travel diary reveals a typically funny and frank moment during her birthday dinner in September at a swank restaurant, just before Abe and Gene's departure on their travels.

"In the evening Dagny, Phil, Gene and his girl, Abe and I all went to the Rôtisserie de la Reine Pédauque and had a tremendous meal as a birthday celebration for me—with so much wine that I had to excuse myself just before the end of the meal to give some of it back to Paris. Didn't feel badly though and thoroughly enjoyed the dinner. "

Eventually the young family returned to England to sail for India on the RMS Strathmore. Unfortunately, Jan no longer kept a travel diary during this part of her journey, or if she did the diary has been lost. It seems clear from letters she wrote later to her family from India that aboard ship the Weisblats were befriended by two young Parsi men from Bombay, Adi Hormasji and Pesy Khan. This led to the family's adoption by a wider Parsi social circle when they reached Bombay.

Parsis (Jan spelled it "Parsee") occupied and still occupy a unique position in Bombay. Parsis are Zoroastrians whose ancestors immigrated to India in the tenth century from Iran. The group is active in Indian society and culture; it has contributed artistic, business, and political leaders. Yet it is always a bit set apart by its own religion, traditions, and ethnic identity. Jan identified strongly with the Parsis' simultaneous love of India and knowledge that they were always going to be defined as "others" by Indian society.

The Parsis they met were enchanted by Jan and Abe's enthusiasm for travel. The couple also represented a novelty to their new friends. Most of the Americans Bombay residents had met had money. Jan and Abe were young people on a budget, firmly in the middle class. Even as Indians rather than Americans the couple would have been unusual. Adi Hormasji and Pesy Khan and their families knew many wealthy people; they were wealthy themselves. They were also familiar with the city's vast underclass, the poor who lined the streets of Bombay. Bombay housed very few people who fell in between the two strata.

When the Strathmore arrived in Bombay, the Weisblats were in for a rude awakening. They had originally planned to be based in the North Indian city of Allahabad. Just before leaving for Europe they had learned that the agricultural institute there was unable to take them. So Abe had written to a colleague and mentor farther south, at Bombay University. He was quickly invited to base his research there and to teach a graduate course at the university.

The funds the Ford Foundation had allotted for living in Allahabad were far from sufficient in the cosmopolitan city of

Bombay, however. The Weisblats stayed at the Taj Mahal Hotel for nearly a month while they looked for accommodations, and they seriously considered having Jan and David return to the United States so that Abe could find simple room and board somewhere.

In the end, their Parsi connections found them a home. Adi Hormasji's friend Feroz Jeejebhoy was a high-level civil servant, a magistrate. Jeej, as he was called, lived in a luxurious three-bedroom apartment in the middle of Bombay and was looking for someone to manage his household and servants. (His wife was staying semi-permanently in England, where their son was studying law.)

In exchange for a minimal rent, the Weisblats enjoyed two of the three bedrooms (each with a bath attached and with a balcony overlooking the city), and Jan threw herself into domestic life in Bombay. She wrote to her parents, "No one could have a more charming host than Mr. Jeejebhoy (or Jeej) who sits by calmly and even seems to enjoy it as we move in, take over, and completely upset his established routine."

Jeej's only request, she later told her family, was that they not move in on a Saturday. His horoscope, drawn shortly after his birth and adhered to throughout his life, stipulated that he must never under any circumstances begin anything important on a Saturday.

At the Jeejebhoy apartment Jan supervised the servants but also cooked a fair amount herself, finding that her Parsi friends wanted to taste American cooking. Macaroni and cheese and pies—apple, lemon meringue, and especially pumpkin—were particular favorites, as well as Southern fried chicken and salad with a French vinaigrette.

Jan's enthusiasm for her life in Bombay bubbles out of the pages of her letters home. Shortly after moving in with Jeej, she wrote to friends back in the States, "I'm sure I'm not a typical Memsahib! I spend at least half the day in the kitchen and I go shopping with the cook at least once a week and take buses instead of taxis—but it's all lots of fun. And people are very kind indeed. No matter where you go, you can feel the friendliness."

The Weisblats not only entertained but were entertained. They became particularly close to Pesy Khan and his family. A wealthy young businessman with a penchant for sports cars, Pesy exhibited a combination of wisdom and innocence that mirrored Jan's own view of the world. In lingering evenings at the Khan and Jeejebhoy homes the friends discussed culture, art, food, and the occult.

The year in India was not without its trials. Like most Americans in the country, all three Weisblats suffered from dysentery from time to time. In late June Jan's letters noted an ominous invasion:

"One of the interesting features of the monsoon has been the onslaught of insect life. We've had cockroaches all the year—but now we are deluged with flies! And since there are no screens on the windows we must wage a constant and, I am afraid, losing battle against them. I noticed that there was a warning against flies in the paper the other day as carriers of typhoid. At least we are happy to have been inoculated and that [David Bruce] has been inoculated!"

Shortly after that the letters home stopped abruptly. Overnight Jan contracted polio and couldn't move her left leg at all. She relocated from Jeej's airy apartment to Bombay's Breach Candy Hospital. (Her Parsi network consisted of doctors as well as lawyers and businessmen.) Later in life she always detested flies, blaming them for spreading the disease.

She never detested Bombay, however. In fact, she always maintained that if she was going to get polio, she was better off getting it in that city than anywhere else. The hospital doctors diagnosed and treated her efficiently. And she knew that Abe and David were well cared for by Mr. Jeejebhoy and the servants, particularly David's ayah, Alice.

A perennially positive person, Jan never doubted that she would get better. Recovery took time, but she did regain most of the use of her bad leg, although she could never again walk for hours or engage in strenuous sports.

And although Abe and her parents insisted that she go back to the United States by plane for therapy as soon as she was able to move, she never doubted that she would return to India.

My mother did indeed come back many times on visits—often meeting artists whose works she and my father collected as the years went by—and eventually spent three years in New Delhi in the 1970s. As she had before she delighted in the colors, the spices, and the people of her beloved India.

That country was always in her heart. When she looked at the art on her walls or threw together a curry or wrote letters to her friends overseas, she remembered the sense of home away from home she had experienced beginning in those months in Bombay.

After a solo trip to Bombay in 1957, my father wrote to her, "A large part of my time in Bombay was spent visiting all our old friends. I had a feeling when I was there that nothing had changed and that it was just as if I was once more sitting in the living room with you, having a chota peg [a little drink] before supper, and not being sure who was going to drop in."

That's how I think of my parents: sitting together sipping a cocktail and looking forward to the next visitor, the next taste, the next experience.

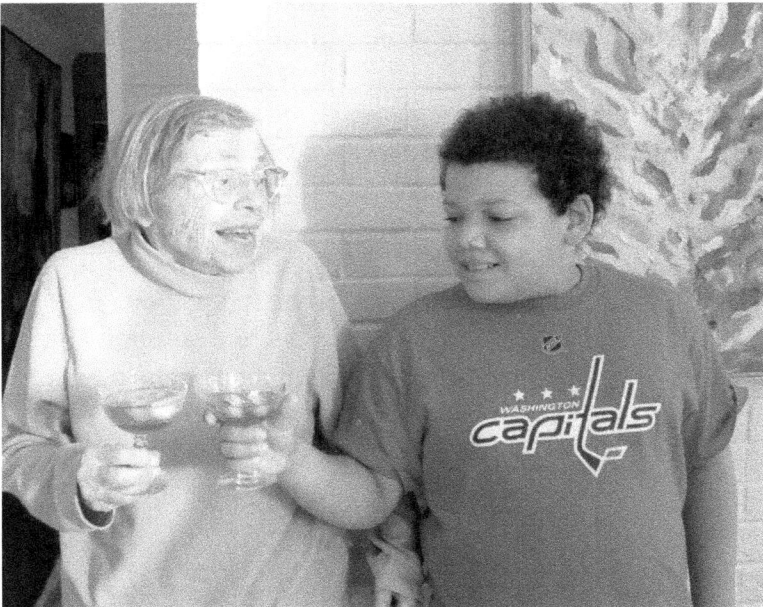

Here Taffy shares a (non-alcoholic!) chota peg with another of her favorite guys, her grandson Michael.

India

by Jan Weisblat

India is an artist's palette,
Strong primary colors against a base of brown.
Brown women in red and gold saris,
Yellow wheat fields waving in the sun,
Emerald tanks below the white-washed village huts
And the tender green of new rice.
Yellow corn lies drying on red roofs in Kulu.
Browns mingle with gray and gold in the Rajasthani desert.
The bright orange-red of the gulmohar
—the flame tree—heralds the spring in Bombay,
And the roof of the world stands white and purple in the
North.
The dhobi spreads his wash of white, yellow, blue and red
On the dull green banks of the river,
And little brown children swim naked
In the green waters of a pond
With their black water buffalo.
India is grey-blue crows in the garden
Shouting a raucous keep-away to other birds,
And sassy black robins flicking red-bellied tails.
The myna birds gather in chattering groups,
Yellow beaks, brown bodies and white tails in flight,
And a tiny green bee-eater sits on my telephone wire.
India is gold sun overhead,
Blue skies in winter,
Yellow skies, heavy with dust, in April and May,
And dark grey monsoon skies
Ready to replenish the parched earth.

August Recipe: Taffy's Chicken Curry

Taffy loved to toss together a simple curry. She used fairly spicy curry powder and ended up with a medium-hot dish.

Ingredients:

a little bit of olive oil or peanut oil
2 chicken breasts, cut in half
1 clove garlic, minced
1 small piece of ginger, minced
1 medium onion, minced
2 heaping teaspoons curry powder
2 heaping teaspoons cumin (use either powdered cumin or slightly crushed cumin seeds)
1 heaping teaspoon chili powder
salt and pepper to taste
2 cups chicken stock
1 small tomato, cut up
1 largish carrot, cut into small coins
the juice of 1 lemon

Instructions:

In a medium sauté pan or Dutch oven heat the oil over medium-high heat; then quickly brown the chicken pieces. Remove them to a plate. Place the garlic, ginger, and onion pieces in the pan. Sauté them until they begin to brown nicely. Sprinkle the curry powder, cumin, chili powder, and salt and pepper over the vegetables. Toss them over medium heat for a minute or two. You don't want them to burn, but you do want them to form a kind of roux.

Pour in a little of the chicken stock to make a paste. Cook the paste for another minute or two; then return the chicken to the pot and add the rest of the stock, along with the tomato. Bring the liquid to a boil, cover the pot, and simmer the curry over low heat for 20 minutes. At the end of the 20 minutes throw in the carrot pieces and simmer the curry for at least 20 minutes longer, still covered. Just before serving stir in the lemon juice.

Serve over rice along with chopped peanuts, coconut, chutney, and yogurt. In our family this serves 4 people. If you have major chicken eaters either plan on serving 2 or double the recipe.

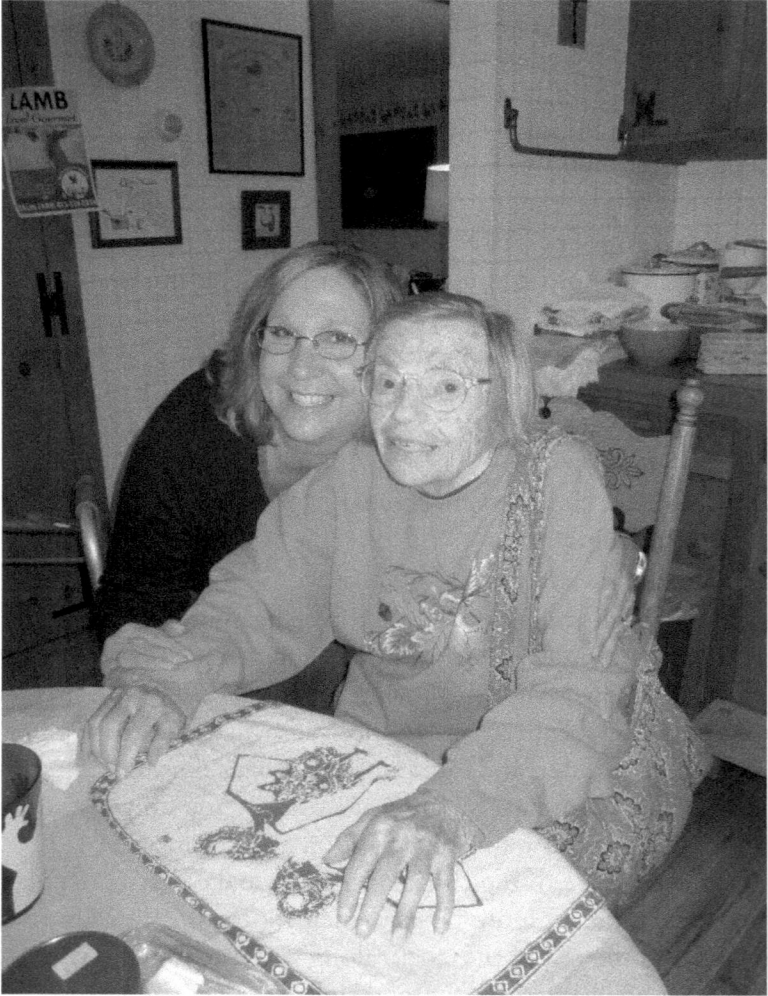

Ready to go out with Pam

SEPTEMBER
Trying to Stay in Place

Thursday, September 8: A Jar over a Candle

Yesterday was quiet in Pudding Hollow.

It had been raining steadily for a couple of days. We still had power. (Hallelujah!) The road was washed out once again in either direction, however, at least for those of us who don't drive big trucks. My mother and I were perforce spending the day at home.

The rain was cooler than last week's so I built a fire in the woodstove. Lorelei Lee, a typical cat, dozed on a rug, as close to the heat as she could get. Taffy and Truffle were stretched out on a couch nearby taking a weather-appropriate nap.

So I had the leisure to think about a topic I had been meaning to address for a couple of weeks: Pat Summitt's recent diagnosis of early-onset dementia.

Patricia Head Summitt, 59, is probably the best known female sports coach in the United States. She may well be the best known coach of either gender. She is widely referred to as the "winningest" coach in college basketball.

During the course of nearly four decades helming the Lady Volunteers at the University of Tennessee (one of my *alma maters*), she has gained a reputation as a fiery yet nurturing teacher and leader.

When she began coaching in 1974 the Lady Vols were an afterthought on the Tennessee athletic scene. Summitt brought her team, and women's basketball in general, into parity and prominence.

Martha Ackmann, the author of a recent biography of pioneering baseball player Toni Stone, wrote an essay last spring that lauded Summitt for her work in promoting gender equality in sports and thereby promoting it in society at large. "The more opportunities we have for women on the courts, the diamonds and athletic fields, the more we challenge stereotypes and move the world forward," Ackmann argued.

The university's athletic director, Joan Cronin, recently summed up Summitt's reputation. "I know what Pat stands for," Cronin said: "excellence, strength, honesty, and courage."

In late August Summitt announced that she had been struggling with cognitive and memory issues for some months. She was diagnosed with dementia late in the spring at the Mayo Clinic.

Her son Tyler and sportswriter Sally Jenkins, a close friend of the coach, helped spread the news of Summitt's diagnosis and her decision to continue coaching the Lady Vols. They explained that changes will be made in the coaching structure. Summitt's able and experienced assistants will take on even more responsibility, particularly during the rush of game time when the head coach's reaction times may suffer. She will continue to do as much as she can for as long as she can, however.

Public reaction to the announcement has been supportive. A Facebook campaign successfully urged fans and supporters throughout the nation to wear orange (the Volunteers' color) a few days after Summitt's announcement.

My friend Bill Dockery, a native Tennessean and a wonderful writer, announced on Facebook that he had hung up a prayer flag of orange "T"s in Summitt's honor. "It won't affect the outcome for Pat—would that it could," wrote Bill, "but it expresses our fear, sadness, empathy, and the hope that acting as a community we can all feel redemption from death and loss."

In general, fellow coaches and the press have praised Summitt's courage in staying on as head coach, although Dan Bernstein of CBS Chicago called for her immediate resignation. He suggested that by keeping her on as head coach the university was violating its "promise to the parents of recruits that their son or daughter is in the best possible hands."

I know that Summitt, her family, her coaching staff, and her athletes face many tough moments in the months and years ahead. My mother was diagnosed with dementia when she was in her 80s—and the doctor who diagnosed it never actually named the disease. By the time Alzheimer's hit her hard, Taffy was too far gone to be aware of, or worried about, the deterioration of her cognitive ability.

For Summitt it is different. It will continue to be different. She is in the prime of her life and her career. She has already taken note of changes in her decision-making process during games as well as in her dealings with her family, friends, and colleagues. These changes will only increase in number with time.

In a moving piece in the *Washington Post* discussing Summitt's diagnosis and decision, Sally Jenkins summed up her own impression of the effects of her friend's illness so far. "There is a faint sense of dimming," wrote Jenkins, "as if a jar has been placed over a candle."

The candle will go on to flicker more and more. Eventually it will be extinguished.

Nevertheless, Bernstein is dead wrong about Summitt's value to the University of Tennessee. The coach's decision to stay on—and the university's unequivocal support of her as ongoing head coach of the Lady Vols—puts her students in the hands of someone who has courage, who can delegate, who asks for no special treatment, and who knows her own worth.

What better hands could those students' parents ask for?

Living with dementia every day as I do, I applaud Summitt's determination to take on yet another leadership role—as a spokeswoman for Alzheimer's awareness—as she continues to inspire and instruct her players.

If she is lucky, basketball will turn out to be for Pat Summitt what music is to my mother: a passionate art that bypasses some of the brain's standard byways and continues to thrive even as dementia takes over much of her world. I wish her this luck, this passion, this clarity.

And I hope her candle will burn on for a long time to come.

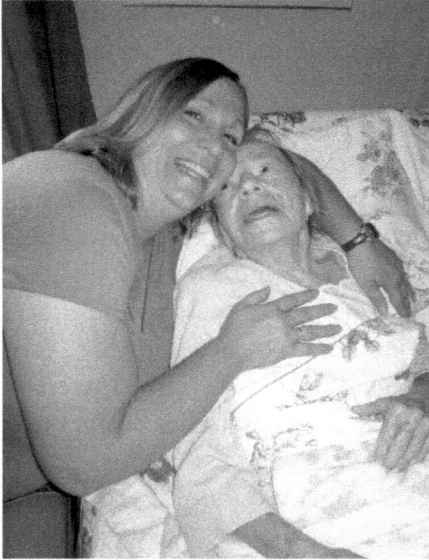

Pam and Taffy in the morning

Friday, September 16: Channeling Sandra Day O'Connor

In 2007 Sandra Day O'Connor's family made a public announcement about her husband. John Jay O'Connor III, who had suffered for many years from Alzheimer's disease, had formed a romantic relationship with a fellow resident of the Phoenix nursing home in which he was living.

Later the former Supreme Court justice elaborated in a question-and-answer session with Deborah Solomon in *The New York Times:*

"He was in a cottage, and there was a woman who kind of attached herself to him. It was nice for him to have someone there who was sometimes holding his hand and to keep him company. And then he was moved to a different cottage, because his condition deteriorated. And in the new cottage, there's another woman who has been very sweet to him. And I'm totally glad."

I recall being intrigued but a little perplexed by Justice O'Connor's reaction. Part of me thought she was being an incredibly good sport. Another part of me couldn't conceive of being able to let go of a spouse so easily after more than five decades of marriage.

I'm not a spouse—but now that I deal with a similar situation as a daughter I have come closer to understanding Sandra Day O'Connor and her marriage.

My mother ADORES her main caregiver here in Massachusetts, Pam Gerry. (Taffy also has Jen Rich, whom she adores almost as much, but Pam comes more often.)

Here's a typical morning scenario.

Taffy lies in bed. I try to get her up, and I'm told "ten more minutes" several times.

Suddenly Pam's voice is heard in the doorway.

Taffy sits upright in bed and says, "You're HERE! I love you, I love you." She happily agrees to wash, get dressed, and eat breakfast … the very activities she has just told me she doesn't want to try.

I usually joke a little at this point, waving at my mother and saying, "Hello! I'm here, too. What am I, chopped liver?"

But I'm actually thrilled for her.

At this point in her life she's a little girl, and I'm her mother figure. She loves me—but she goes through many less than ecstatic moments with me when I have to ask her to take her pills … or do a few exercises … or wait a few minutes to go outside into the sunshine.

In contrast, Pam is her friend, her pal, her playmate. Everything Pam does is designed to make life more fun for Taffy. And Taffy blossoms in Pam's company.

They do puzzles and craft projects. They read books. They giggle together. They go out for ice cream. Last week they took a trip to the County Fair to play bingo, view giant pumpkins, and stroke lambs.

Like Sandra Day O'Connor with her husband, I'm "totally glad" that my mother sometimes prefers someone else to me. It's a gift to both of us that she can find someone perfect to play with at this point in her life. More than ever before, more than anything else, she needs joy in her life. And her joy makes me joyful.

It's odd but strangely encouraging that her second childhood is helping me to grow up at last.

Friday, September 23: Ordering In

My friend Jennifer went to cooking school in New York City more than 20 years ago. She returned home with excellent culinary skills—and an enormous appreciation of the convenience of life in the Big Apple.

"You can get absolutely anything or any service delivered to your door there," she told me, recalling waking up in the morning and calling for someone to bring her a bagel, a cup of coffee, and a newspaper instead of venturing outside her apartment door.

Recently I've realized that, thanks to the internet and to a few people who love to help others, Hawley, Massachusetts, is approaching New York in terms of convenience.

We can't actually get bagels delivered here. We can't even buy real bagels nearby. And don't get me started on good Chinese food.

(Don't feel too sorry for us. We have darling New York friends who occasionally serve as our bagel-delivery service.)

Nevertheless, we do now receive a number of goods and services I wouldn't have imagined we could get in our remote hamlet—goods and services that make life with a frail person who has dementia much easier.

I do a huge amount of shopping for Taffy on the internet. Several things I have looked for in vain at local stores (even medical supply stores) have winged their way toward us courtesy of Amazon.com and other web sites.

These include a thermometer that goes into the ear rather than the mouth, waterproof pillowcases, and a raised toilet seat.

Some things I can get only by going to Greenfield, our county seat, are cheaper and quicker (since I don't drive to Greenfield often) when ordered online. I have a regular monthly order for disposable underwear from Amazon. I don't even have to carry it into the house since our UPS man is very obliging.

Even more useful than the goods coming to our house are the people. We have two in particular who have hit it off with Taffy.

Bev LaBelle, who works part time in a beauty salon in Greenfield, goes to several elderly clients a month with a service she calls "Totally Toes." She chats with Taffy, soaks and massages the maternal feet, inspects them for any problems, and clips toenails—all with much more fun and convenience (and for much less money) than a podiatrist.

Samantha Thompson, who works in a beauty salon in Shelburne Falls, goes two days a week to private clients in their homes to do their hair. As recently as last year, an outing to get her hair cut made Taffy happy. Now she is so tired and confused that going to the beauty shop in town wears her out completely.

Samantha calmly and gently cuts her elderly clients' hair (and anyone else's—Pam and I had ours trimmed recently as well!). Taffy was asleep half the time Samantha worked on her the other day, which didn't seem to faze this young woman a bit. Best of all, Samantha travels with her two cute daughters, four-year-old Gracie and six-month-old Olivia. Nothing engages my mother like small children.

Like Bev, Samantha is reasonable in price and pleasant to have in the house. They both brighten my mother's day … and lighten my load.

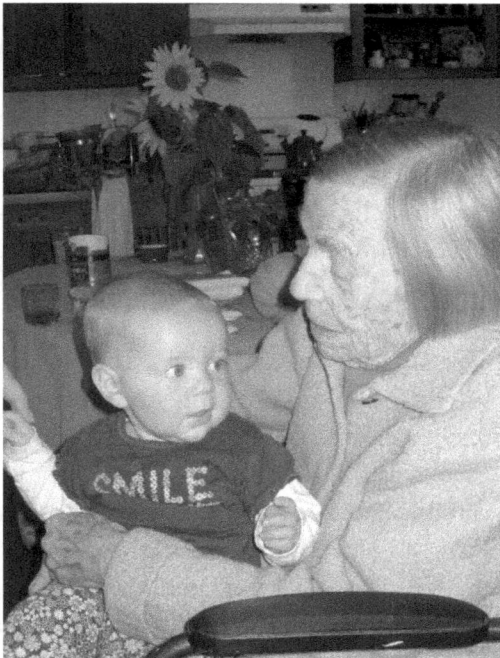

Taffy with a special visitor

Thursday, September 29: Road Closed

Our main road to town, Route 8A north, was suddenly closed this morning—inconveniencing and frustrating most folks here in Pudding Hollow, our small section of Hawley, Massachusetts.

We have become accustomed to the constant road construction that followed Hurricane Irene. Nevertheless, the decision to close the road for at least two to three days, made late yesterday and announced haphazardly only to people who were driving by just then, has flummoxed us a bit.

Today people are forced to get to us via Route 8A from the south. That road is technically closed (and is definitely iffy in many spots) but can be traveled if one is careful. The travel just takes a LOT longer.

Our hospice aide, our hospice nurse, and our home aide (the fabulous Pam) all said they were coming this morning.

Pam is the only one who actually made it—and even then travel took her almost two hours (she lives only 15 minutes away under normal circumstances) because an accident on one of the alternate routes forced her to try yet another alternate route.

The other two drove around for quite a while and then gave up. I don't blame them.

Our twisty, muddy road has symbolic meaning for me right now. I am beginning to see "road closed" signs on my mother's body and mind as well. Her path to better health isn't completely closed, but it is certainly getting rocky. Getting places, literally and figuratively, seems to take her such a long time that she may decide to give up.

She is increasingly tired and weak. The hospice people, who originally thought she would probably not stay on with them, have begun to describe her symptoms as typical of the end of life.

I don't know why I'm surprised by this. Taffy is 93, she is frail, and she's confused. Surprised I am, however, just as I have always been when Taffy has taken a turn for the worse.

Part of me still thinks of her as my ever strong, iron-willed, eternally healthy mother. In all probability that part of me will continue to see her that way long after she dies.

Deep down in her essence she is that person. She certainly still exhibits the will of her youth from time to time. Nevertheless, she has been hit by forces as relentless in their own way as a hurricane—and her road becomes rougher by the day.

Our patterns are gradually changing. She sleeps more and is more agitated when she can't sleep. She uses her walker less and her wheelchair more. She often needs more than one person to get her up or put her to bed. (She is apt to slide right down to the floor if not carefully handled.)

Her caregivers and I have determined that transporting her back to be near my brother and his family in Virginia, which we planned to do sometime this fall, would exhaust her little body and confuse her mind further. My brother is coming for a visit next week, and I'm sure he and his wife and son will come again when they can. Meanwhile, we are enjoying the company of friends, neighbors, and caregivers here in Massachusetts ... when they can get to us!

Happily, the animals are always around to snuggle.........

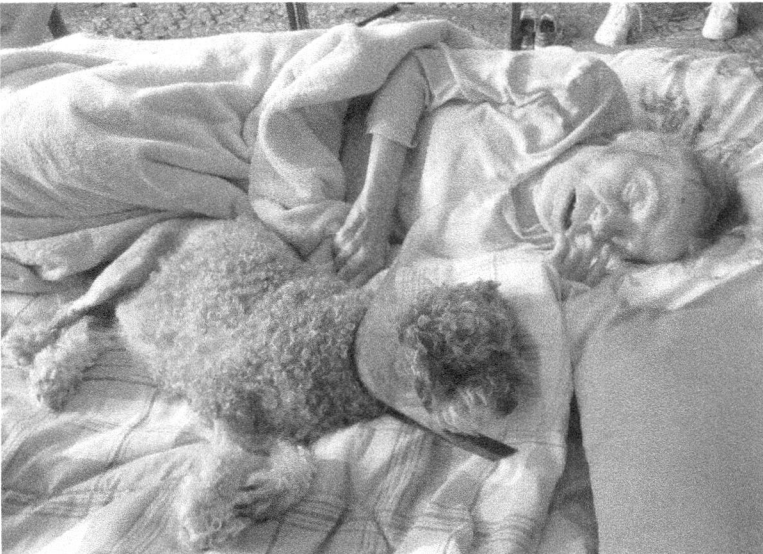

September Meditation: Taffy at Work

Taffy spent most of her early working years as an elementary-school teacher, attending the Bank Street School in New York and then going on to teach wherever she was—New Jersey, Washington, Wisconsin, the Philippines, India. As the years went by she began to use her extensive command of French more and more in her teaching; in the late 1960s she received a master's degree in French literature from Seton Hall University.

She loved teaching at just about any level. The seventh graders in our international school in India were the bane of most teachers' existence, but not of Taffy's. If their hormones caused them to act up, she would draw herself up to her full five-foot, one-and-one-half-inch height and bellow at them in her deep voice. Then she would laugh … and they would smile and calm down.

She took a few years off from work when my brother and I were very small, although I wouldn't precisely call her a stay-at-home mom during that period. She volunteered extensively (her favorite cause was the local Y.W.C.A.) and acted in many amateur dramatic productions. She had always adored theater but never got to play the lead in plays in high school. As an adult she finally got to play her favorite role, Kate in *The Taming of the Shrew.*

In her 50s Taffy changed careers and went into the antique business in western Massachusetts, starting a seasonal shop called Charlemont House Gallery with her friend Claire Roth in the back of Claire's house in Charlemont. Claire was tall and slender; Taffy, short and plump. Despite their physical incongruities they had much in common.

They had similar streaks of practicality and parallel senses of humor. They also had complementary knowledge about antiques. Claire knew all there was to know about Oriental rugs and Victorian furnishings; Taffy specialized in dining-room items such as pressed glass and Staffordshire china. The enterprise gave them a great deal of satisfaction. It gave their children a lot of fun, too. I recall playing cards, making salads, and helping refinish furniture with the partners and with Claire's daughters Amy and Lyzz.

When Claire retired to take a full-time job in New York, Taffy kept the business going for another 20 years. She moved to the nearby village of Shelburne Falls and christened the business the Merry Lion after Mary Lyon, the founder of Mount Holyoke.

The shop was many things to her—a vehicle for lifelong learning (she adored taking classes about antiques and appraisal), a place in which to cultivate new and old friends, and to some extent a source of income. (I have a feeling she would have kept the place open even if it hadn't made a penny.)

After Claire's retirement Taffy found a new partner—folk-artist Judith Russell, who turned the whole shop into a gallery and play room. The Merry Lion looked out on the Bridge of Flowers in Shelburne Falls, and Judy produced many views of the bridge while seated at her painter's desk in the shop.

Judy and Taffy attracted an odd but charming assortment of visitors and customers to the shop. One summer a dowser developed a crush on Judy and stopped by almost daily to discuss his trade. Artists, playwrights, tourists, and carpenters visited the shop to look at merchandise and occasionally purchase it.

The conversation in the Merry Lion was always lively, and so was the decor. My mother and Judy decked the shop out for every conceivable holiday, always giving the papier-mâché lion in the shop window something to wear that suited the season.

They were particularly proud when they received a note from Bill Clinton (then a presidential candidate) thanking them for their red, white, and blue "Vote for Clinton/Gore" display.

As you can probably tell from the description above, my mother's place of business was never just about business. It fused public and private seamlessly, bringing a sense of home and play into the workplace. Customers responded to the warmth of the shop, the enthusiasm of the shopkeepers, and the occasional edible treats given out at the Merry Lion.

Taffy retired in her early 80s to spend more time with her sole grandchild, my nephew Michael. She enjoyed her life of relative leisure (she was busy even at home) but occasionally directed a slightly wistful glance toward the building that had housed her shop.

I directed a few such glances myself. At work as at home Taffy set a strong example for me.

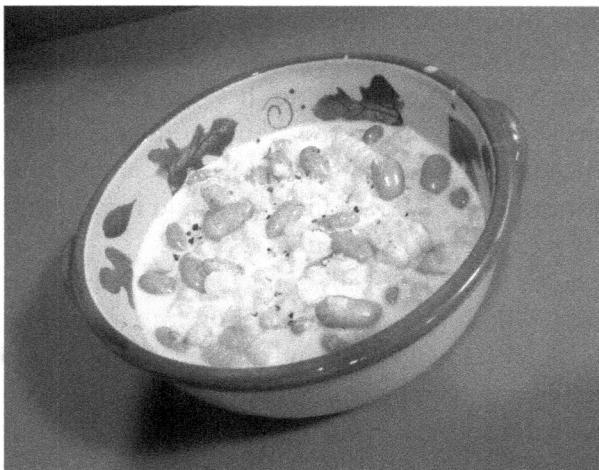

September Recipe: Taffy's Succotash

Each year that I can remember Taffy kept her eyes open in August and September for what she called "pink beans." They are also known as cranberry beans; when I purchased them at Foster's Supermarket the autumn after her death they were labeled simply "shell beans."

These fresh beans are encased in pink-and-white-mottled skins. When removed from their shells the beans themselves are also white with pink flecks, although they trade those colors for a less exciting uniform beige when cooked.

Whenever my mother saw them, she would purchase them, take them home, and make succotash. I have a feeling the beans were grown on her grandparents' farm when she was growing up because they represented home to her. After a lifetime of watching her cook and eat them, I find that they speak of home to me as well.

Taffy never actually measured the beans or the corn or the cream so the quantities that follow are approximate. If you want to dress up your succotash, add a little sautéed onion, some herbs, and/or a little bacon garnish. My mother never did so my recipe is rather plain.

Its flavor is far from plain, however. The beans have a subtle but unmistakable nutty taste that always reminds me of my slightly nutty mother. When you throw in the corn and the cream (or half and half) and grind a small hill of pepper on top you end up with a dish fit for a queen.

The succotash embodies my mother's ability to take joy in simple, everyday pleasures. If I can be half as joyful in my lifetime, I will count myself lucky.

Ingredients:

2 cups shelled cranberry beans
2 cups water, plus more water as needed
salt to taste
the cooked kernels from 3 ears of corn
cream or half and half as needed (between 1/2 cup and 1 cup)
lots of freshly ground pepper

Instructions:

Pick over the beans, removing any that have turned brown.

In a medium saucepan bring the cranberry beans, water, and salt to a boil. Reduce the heat, and simmer until the beans are tender but not mushy. This will take between 15 and 45 minutes, depending on the age of the beans. (The younger they are, the less time it will take.)

Stir the beans from time to time while they simmer, and be sure to add more water if you need to. At the end of the simmering process the beans should still have a little—but not a lot of—liquid in their pan. Do not drain off this liquid.

Stir in the corn and cream or half and half. The beans should be in a gentle liquid bath but shouldn't be drowning. Cook for another 5 minutes or so, until everything is heated through.

Grind pepper over the succotash and serve. Serves 6 to 8 hearty eaters.

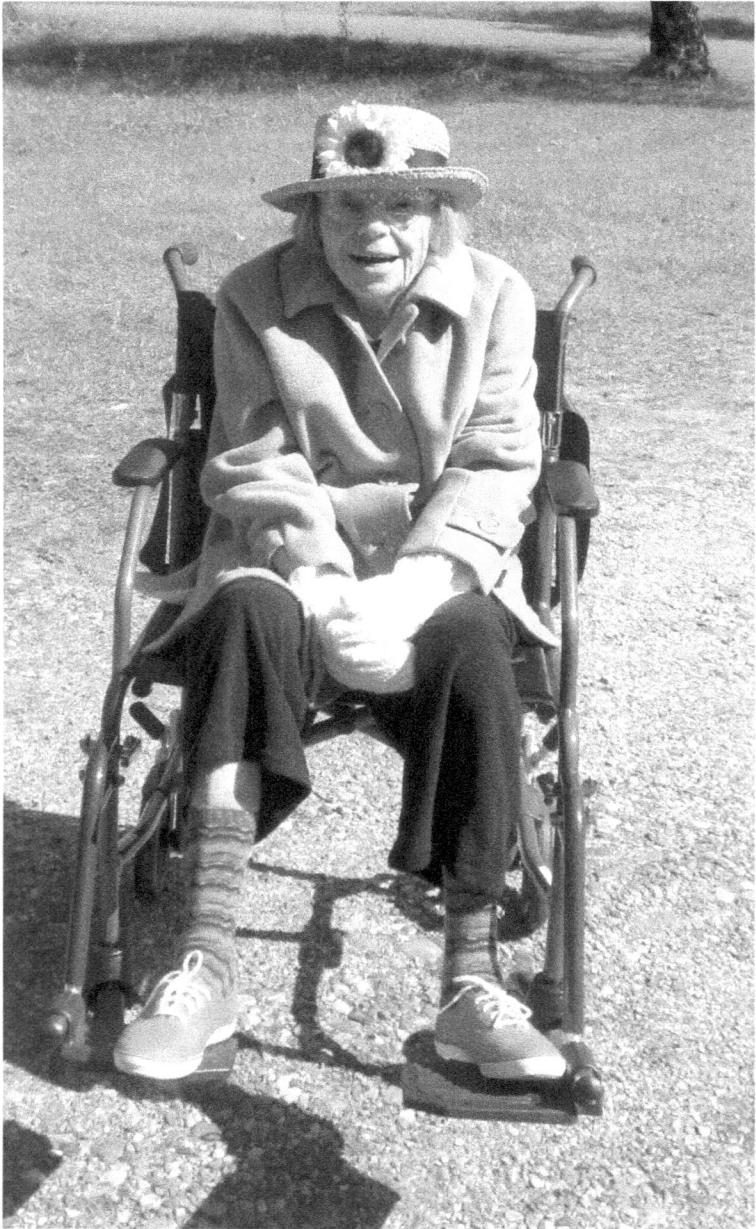

OCTOBER
Darkening Skies

Friday, October 7: Let the Sunshine In!

I have noted before that Taffy and I specialize in short-term memories.

She remembers things only in the short term because of her dementia. I remember them that way because that's the nature of my brain. It always has been.

That short-term bias has made the weather difficult for us for much of the past few weeks.

A normal person would say that it had rained a lot.

To the two of us—particularly to my mother—it seemed as though it had rained FOREVER.

One of our hospice aides told me that she believes that people near the end of their lives lose consciousness of the sun.

I strongly disagree with this view. I have known a lot of people who have died in the fall, just as it starts to get darker and darker. And I have known even more who have died in the early winter.

Technically, the sun starts rising earlier and higher right after December 21. Nevertheless, most of us in northern climes feel that dull ache in January when it seems as though the cold and the darkness will never recede. I can see how people barely hanging on to life could give up hope in January—or even in October.

Taffy's spirits dipped during the rainy days. She would look out the window frequently, clearly hoping to catch a glimpse of a little brightness. And then she would lie down and go to sleep.

Suddenly on Wednesday we started to see the sun. Yesterday was an ideal fall day. Clouds barely laced its deep blue sky. And its sunshine was pure gold.

Now my little Energizer Bunny mother has become almost manic.

She gets cold when she goes outdoors in her wheelchair even when it seems warm to the rest of us; she has taken to going out in a coat and mittens. Nevertheless, out she goes, with her faithful dog trotting by her side.

If she's too tired to go out, she sits in the living room, which was designed to catch maximum sun during the fall and winter months. Sometimes she reads a simple book with Pam or listens to me sing. More often she just alternates between dozing and looking at the light on the fall leaves.

She's not strong. She's definitely confused. Even so, she still gets as much pleasure as she can out of each ray of sunshine.

Friday, October 14: Until She Isn't

At one point when my mother was in the hospital in August my brother and I asked the nurse who had just come on duty to update us on our mother's status. She hadn't treated Taffy before so she consulted Taffy's file on the computer.

"This is adorable," she told us. "It says here that your mother is 'pleasantly demented.'"

"She is," I replied. "Until she isn't."

What I meant, as I have indicated in these pages before, is that from time to time SOMETHING—an infection or bad weather or a little change in the dementia—can make even my cute little mother difficult to live with.

She has been going through one of her "until she isn't" phases this past week. Most of the time she's just fine, but she has had several nights of sleeplessness (and she and I do love our sleep) and several episodes of restlessness and anger.

She even yelled at her aide, Pam (she NEVER yells at Pam), when Pam tried to keep her from giving chocolate to the dog.

Taffy's aides, the hospice nurses, and I are working to diagnose this behavior. It may stem from one of her standard urinary-tract infections. She is now beginning a course of antibiotics. If she starts to feel better, we will know we have a diagnosis.

On the other hand, the nurses think that she may be also be suffering from end-of-life delirium. This condition has its own nuances.

If Taffy IS suffering from delirium, it sounds as though the best solution is anti-psychotic medication. This makes me nervous.

Don't get me wrong: I want my mother to be her happy self again. I hate giving her drugs, however. The antibiotics last for only a week or ten days. The anti-psychotic drugs could be in use for a long time.

If she takes too few drugs, she could still be sleepless and unhappy. If she takes too many, Taffy could lose her spirit. That spirit is precious not just to us caregivers but to her immediate family, friends, other relatives, and neighbors.

I'm sure we'll learn how to deal with Taffy's restlessness in time. Nevertheless, it amazes me that just when I think I have figured out how to handle my mother's illness it takes a new course.

Taffy always liked to challenge her children. Now she's doing it without even trying.

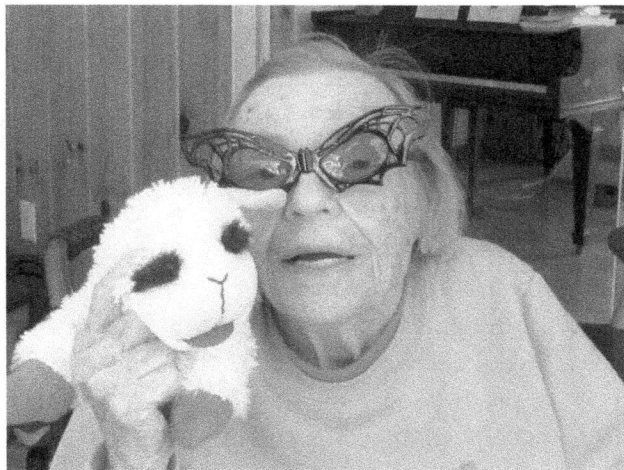

Taffy looks quite contrary wearing my spider-web glasses. (I have no idea what Lamb Chop is doing in this picture.)

Tuesday, October 25: Gingerbread and Applesauce

On Saturday my mother's sister Lura came to lunch with three of her children. My brother David was already visiting with his family so the table was crowded and spirited. Taffy looked a little astonished to have so much company … and she dozed off frequently. Nevertheless, she appeared pleased with the group and popped into the conversation from time to time.

When we were planning my aunt's visit her son David and his wife Mardi told me that they would bring gingerbread to go with the applesauce I always have in the house. This winning food combination paid tribute to a book my mother wrote in her 50s titled *Gingerbread and Applesauce*.

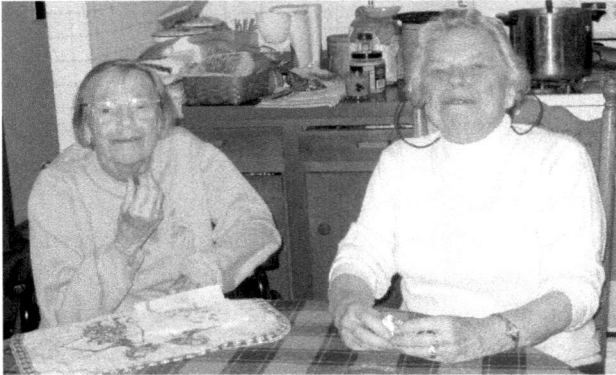

Sisters share a nosh of gingerbread.

This memoir shares her recollections of her parents' younger lives as they were related to her. In my own copy, originally my grandmother's, my grandmother Clara carefully inscribed a few corrections about dates, people, and places. I treasure that double connection to my family's history.

I never asked Taffy why she chose the title "Gingerbread and Applesauce." Unfortunately, it is too late now for her to articulate a response to that question.

I would guess that she saw her family story as the sort of classic, wholesome American fare that those two dishes represent, individually and together. She also ate both foods frequently at her mother's and grandmothers' tables so they literally represented a taste of the past to her.

Taffy always presented herself as a rather plain, straightforward person just as she thought of gingerbread and applesauce as plain, straightforward foods. These dishes have never been precisely plain, however. Nor has my mother.

Like Taffy, the apple trees in our yard from which I make sauce are complex, picturesque, and unpredictable. In years like this they produce more apples than we can gather. In others they offer only their silhouette along the horizon for nourishment. These trees have been here longer than I can remember, and their gnarly beauty reflects their age and character.

Also like Taffy, gingerbread is chock full of surprises, including its signature spices and its deep vein of molasses.

Taffy may have thought of herself as simple, but she went beyond her WASPy New England girlhood in many ways, revealing her own special flavors.

Her marriage to my father was not only a love match but a tribute to her adventurous spirit. To her, a Jewish boy from New York was exotic. She fought for their right to marry. And she fought for him—and occasionally with him—throughout their 53-year marriage. She adored lost causes, the literal and figurative spices of India, the language and architecture of France, and her many and varied friends.

One of my favorite Taffy stories comes from the early days of her marriage, when she and my father were living in a tiny studio apartment in the District of Columbia. He worked for the U.S. Department of Agriculture; she, for the French Mission for Industrial Production. (I may have this name wrong; it was a trade organization of some sort.)

My father traveled a lot on business. When he was away Taffy frequently invited her friend and protégé Edward to sleep on the couch. Edward was often in need of a place to stay. A musical young man from Florida, Edward was witty and charming and intensely vulnerable. Most of his friends were aware that he was gay. In the 1940s he was reluctant to admit it, even to himself.

One evening Taffy threw a cocktail party to which some of her French coworkers were invited. Edward played bartender.

"Is that your husband, Janice?" asked her boss in French.

"Mais non," she replied. She pointed to a photograph of my absent father. "This is my husband. That one [gesturing toward Edward] just sleeps here." She smiled mysteriously.

Before that evening Taffy had been thought of in her office as a naïve, puritanical New Englander. From then on she was regarded as one of the most cosmopolitan Americans her sophisticated French colleagues had met.

She was tickled by her newfound reputation even though she would never have dreamed of being unfaithful to my father.

My mother was, and remains, a wholesome yet spicy helping of gingerbread and applesauce.

Monday, October 31: All Hallow's Eve

Yesterday our neighbor Alice remarked that we had been celebrating Halloween for more than a month in the Weisblat household.

She had a point.

Alas, we have had only one trick or treater in the entire time we have lived in our home in Hawley, Massachusetts. We're too remote. The little children who live around the corner ("around the corner" is a mile and a half away) go to community parties or wander through the next big town in search of treats. Our neighborhood just isn't dense enough to make the effort of going from door to door worthwhile.

Nevertheless, to paraphrase Ebenezer Scrooge's pronouncement about another holiday, we honor Halloween in our hearts here ... and in our home.

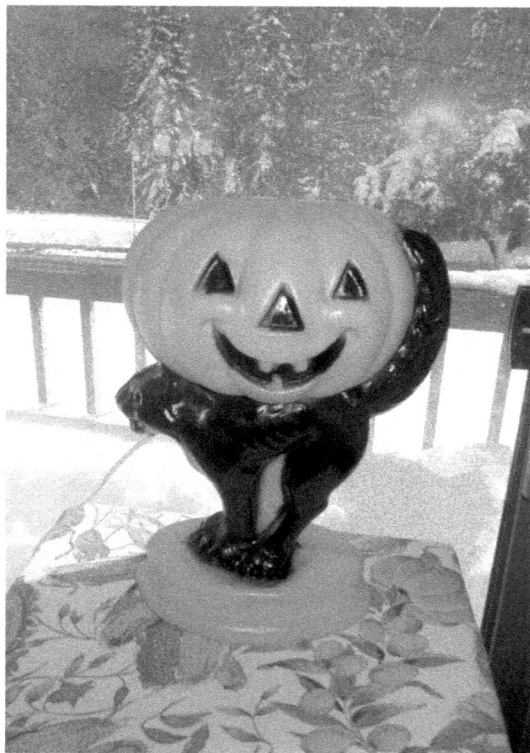

We have been using our Halloween dinnerware (melamine—don't hate me!) for weeks now. Lights are strewn in and out of doors, and spooky miniature houses light up the evening. This year's newest purchase, a salad-server set that looks like skeletal hands and arms, adorns the orange-and-black-covered table whether we are eating salad or not.

Truffle has TWO Halloween costumes: she alternates between fairy-princess and turtle modes. (She also has a bright orange sweatshirt for the cold weather so she can look a bit like a pumpkin.) Taffy and I don't go in for costumes, but we do sport accessories such as haunted-house socks, spooky sunglasses, and devil horns.

This year nature decided to get into the act and dress up as Christmas for Halloween. The snow is lovely, but I'm happy to say that it is melting relatively quickly.

I have always adored Halloween. Being short, I dressed up and meandered from door to door each October 31 into my college years. I loved the candy. I loved the magic and mystery of the night even more.

Halloween is a time at which people both celebrate and transcend boundaries—boundaries between fall and winter, light and dark, fantasy and reality, life and death. It's fun and scary, frivolous and powerful.

All Hallows' Eve is even more precious to me this year because it seems to symbolize my personal situation with my mother. We're on the cusp of her darkness, her death. I don't try to deny that reality. In her own way neither does Taffy. The words "death" and "dying" have been coming up in her muddled conversation a lot lately, as if she is attempting to process this stage of her life to the best of her ability.

Nevertheless, I try to make the most of each experience we share, of the momentary flexibility of the boundaries that confront us. When Taffy is awake (and she is sleeping more and more) we enjoy the orange lights, the woodstove, the camaraderie of friends, and a little spooky music.

We don't rage against the dying of the light. But we do light a lot of candles.

October Meditation: Aunt Jerusha and Community

My mother always loved acting. I inherited the thick slice of ham in my nature from her, although she was always better at creating characters than I. Any character I play is a version of me.

She in turn inherited her love of theatrics from her father, Bruce Hallett. My uncle, Bruce Junior, still recalls sitting at his homework and listening to his father and sister discuss (and recite!) Portia's dissertation on mercy from *The Merchant of Venice*:

> *The quality of mercy is not strain'd,*
> *It droppeth as the gentle rain from heaven*
> *Upon the place beneath: it is twice blest;*
> *It blesseth him that gives and him that takes....*

Taffy performed in numerous plays in high school. She was thwarted from playing romantic leads then by her youth—she had skipped a grade in elementary school—and by the presence of future Broadway and film star Teresa Wright at Columbia High School. Nonetheless, Taffy earned some plum roles, playing the Wicked Witch of the West in *The Wizard of Oz* and the lead role in the story of Aladdin.

In college Taffy blossomed as an accomplished amateur thespian in French as well as English. And she was active in community theater throughout her young married life. One of her scrapbooks includes a 1959 newspaper clipping about an upcoming production of the Library Players in East Orange, New Jersey.

It reads, "Jan Weisblat, who has been in all of the productions to date, will play a prominent part. Her ability to mirror and mime the actions of blowsy ladies, stern housekeepers, prim wives and flippity females [has] made her a natural for all of the East Orange Library Players' productions."

When Hawley, Massachusetts, the site of her summer home, prepared to celebrate its 1992 bicentennial, Taffy naturally volunteered to participate in the pageant honoring the town's history.

Like most of the cast, she played a couple of different roles in addition to lending her low if limited singing voice to the chorus of the pageant. (Hawley is not a large town.)

Her most prominent and favorite role was that of one of the town's true mothers, Jerusha King (1788-1882). Aunt Jerusha, as she was called, was a well known citizen of her day. Educated at home, she served as the town's first historian. She passed down the few stories about Hawley's early days we have today, including the tale of Hawley's first Thanksgiving.

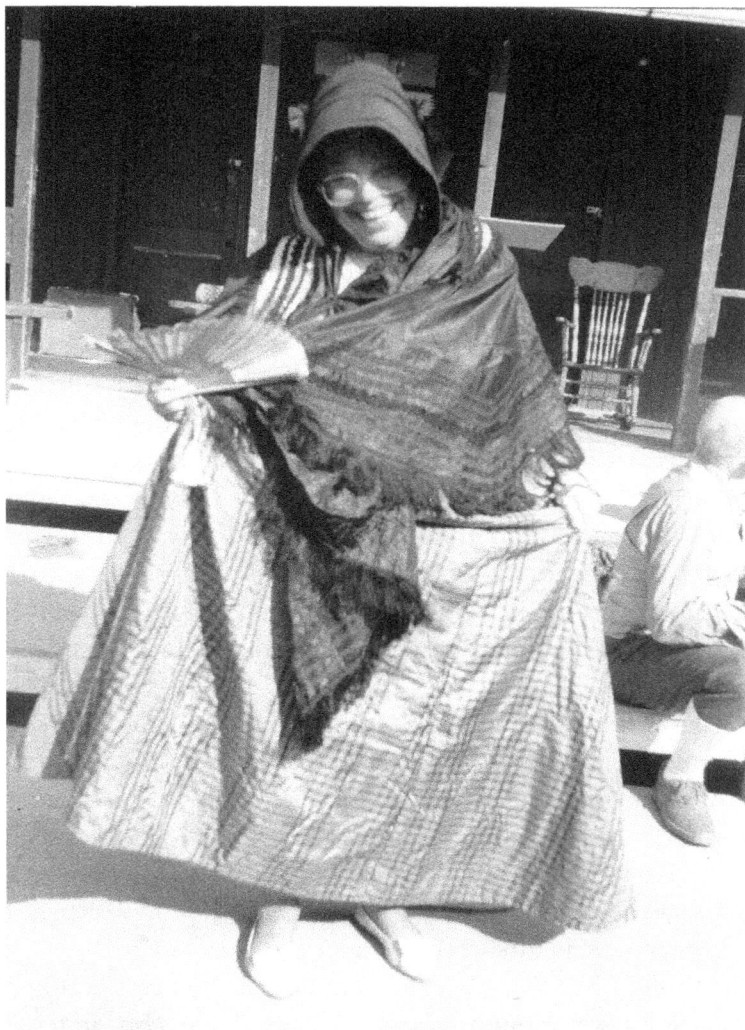

Aunt Jerusha in costume

One obituary recalled, "She was possessed of a fine constitution, was active and industrious, and for many long years 'Aunt' Jerusha's hospitality was extended to friends. Her name was a household word and she was one of those town aunts who is a friend to everybody."

Aunt Jerusha/Taffy appeared in the pageant in a scene in which confused courting couples are sorted out by Jerusha and her best friend Lucy Hitchcock. Lucy was played by Charlotte Thwing, a darling Hawley resident who was a bit older than Taffy but shared with my mother a love of fun and a spirit of eternal youth. "Lucy" didn't always remember her lines or her blocking, but the scene-stealing Jerusha kept her on the straight and narrow with extemporaneous dialogue and, when necessary, tiny shoves.

Their scene together was a delight, as was the entire pageant. It summed up not only much of Hawley's history but also the sense of togetherness we have always felt in this small hilltown.

Throughout Taffy's final year, and even before that year when I was taking care of her, I found myself eternally grateful for the community around us. Neighbors stopped by all the time to help out or just to visit. (Even in her final days my mother enjoyed company!) Our minister, Cara, came to see Taffy at least once a week. And we received phone calls, food, and flowers all the time.

One day in 2010, in her infatuation with the autumn sun, Taffy made an unauthorized break from the house with her walker. I thought she was napping until the town road crew showed up at the door.

"Your mother seems to be hiking to Charlemont," Wayne Clark told me in his laconic drawl. When I found my mother she was WAY down the road chatting unrepentantly with a man she had found while walking. (Believe me, it's not easy to find stray men in Hawley!)

"I knew you'd find me," she said with a big grin on her face. I had to grin back as I thanked the man and the road crew.

Looking back on this and similar experiences, I am still grateful for the community around Taffy. I am also grateful to Taffy/Jan herself, and to my father, Abe. What I saw during Taffy's performance as Aunt Jerusha, and what I now realize I saw for most of my life, was a model for building a sense of community.

Like most small New England towns, Hawley can be a little insular. "New people" and "summer people" take a while to get accepted. My parents never pretended to be descended from the town's first families, and they were never pushy about their desire to be a part of the town.

Instead, they slowly made themselves at home in Hawley. They asked questions. They volunteered to help with sales and events. They brought small gifts to children. They cooked and baked. (Well, my mother cooked and baked. My father was not a cook or a baker.) They smiled. They laughed. They listened.

With each bowl of soup, each question answered, each smiling performance, they made a place for themselves in town. By the time Taffy needed Hawley to give something back to her (and to me), she had no need to ask for help. She and I were cradled by our hills and by their inhabitants.

I am still cradled by Hawley—and when I stray from its boundaries I still seem to find community without even thinking about it, thanks to my parents' example. They worked to sustain the notions of home and community wherever they went in this country and abroad. And they were repaid over and over again for that work.

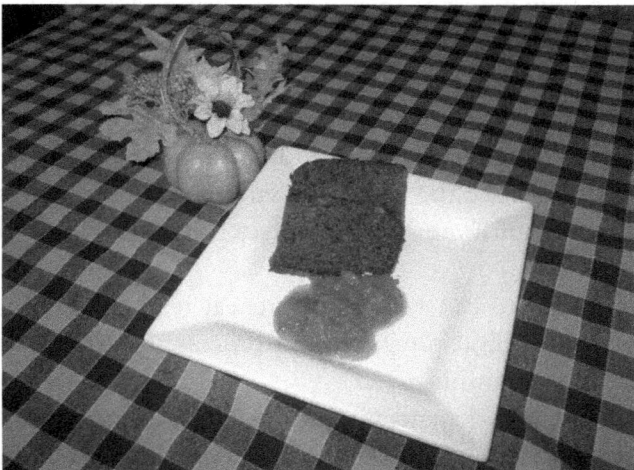

Gingerbread and Applesauce

October Recipe: Windfall Applesauce

Taffy and I liked to make this sauce from the trees in our front yard, although we usually included a few apples from a local orchard as well for variety.

Ingredients:

enough apples to make 6 generous cups of cut-up apples (preferably more than 1 variety)
1 cinnamon stick
1 pinch salt
1/4 cup sweet apple cider, plus additional cider as needed
maple syrup to taste, depending on the tartness of your apples (1 to 2 tablespoons should suffice)

Instructions:

Wash the apples and quarter them (actually, I tend to cut them into eighths if they are at all big). Remove any bad spots, but don't worry about cutting out the core and seeds if you have a food mill.

Place the apple pieces, the cinnamon stick, the salt, and the cider in a 4-quart pot. Bring the mixture to a simmer over low heat, covered, and simmer it until the apples soften, checking frequently to see whether you need to add more cider to keep the sauce from burning. The cooking time will depend on the type and age of your apples and how many of them you are using. A 6-cup batch may take as little as 25 minutes, but a larger, firmer batch can take up to an hour.

Let the apples cool for a few minutes; then run them through a food mill. Discard the skin and seeds (excellent pig food or compost!), and place the sauce in a saucepan. Add maple syrup to taste, and heat until the syrup dissolves, stirring to keep the syrup from burning.

If you want to can your sauce, reheat it to the boiling point, ladle it into sterilized pint jars, and process the jars in a boiling-water bath for 20 minutes.

The yield will depend on your apples. Six generous cups of apple pieces provide about 1 pint of sauce. Feel free to multiply this recipe if your apple harvest is copious.

NOVEMBER
Home and Thanksgiving

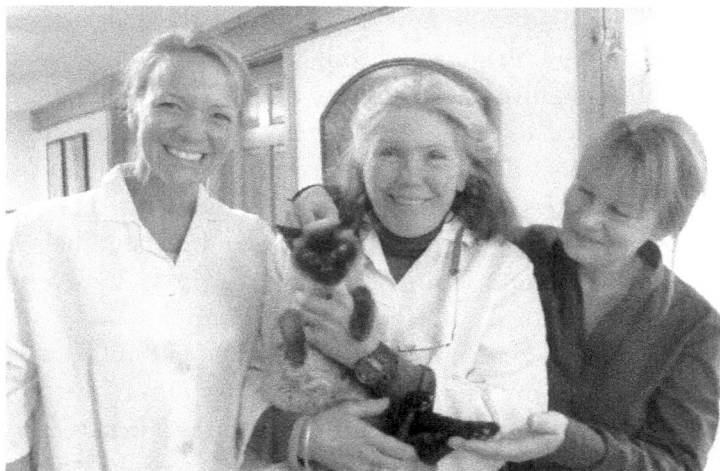

Lorelei Lee with part of her care team
From left to right: Heather, Tori, and Sayward

Tuesday, November 8: Moving Toward Kitty Hospice

Last week it looked as though we were heading for a second hospice situation in our house. Luckily, we seem to have averted it ... for the present.

Tuesday evening Lorelei Lee, our 20-year-old Siamese cat, started acting weird. Her digestive system underwent frequent crises. And suddenly she could neither straighten out her body nor curl into her usual napping ball. She was sort of permanently arched—and not very happy.

She tried in vain to flatten herself to sit under the woodstove. At bedtime she found herself unable to nestle in the crook of my arm (her favorite sleeping position). She settled for crouching over me and resting her head rather sadly on my shoulder. If she could have sighed, she would have.

In the morning I called her vet's office. Lorelei Lee has been a patient of Victoria Howell since LL was a kitten and Tori was just establishing her practice. We have all grown up together. Gale, one of Tori's helpers, fit LL and me into the schedule.

At the office Tori and her staff gathered around Lorelei in concern. Tyrone, one of the office cats, tried to kiss her.

I had been aware that my cat was getting skinnier by the day, but I hadn't realized quite how much weight she had lost. When we put her on the scale she weighed in at 3.8 pounds ... down from more than 12 pounds in her plump prime.

Tori suggested injecting Lorelei with fluids and running tests on her organs. She also recommended an appetite pill and some new high-calorie food that could be mixed with the cat's normal bland diet. (The poor thing has been on bland diet and baby food for months on account of her tendency to throw up every few hours when fed anything at all challenging.)

I have mentioned before that giving Lorelei pills is no easy task. I warned Tori that my cat was likely to wet her during the process, but she decided to take the risk. Ironically, Lorelei behaved herself when Tori and Robin popped the pill into her mouth. It was only when Robin returned the ailing creature to my lap that the urine gushed forth. Lorelei may have been sickly, but she still had her wits about her ... and she clearly knew who had approved the pill giving.

Tori lent me some deodorizing spray (my jeans smelled pretty awful) and sent us home with a promise to report back on the tests the next day.

To make a long story short, the tests proved reasonably promising. Lorelei's organs are a little down, but they're not out. Her back has regained its flexibility. And she has responded beautifully to the new food and the fluids.

In fact, she is doing so well on the fluids that Tori had me come back yesterday to learn how to inject them into my kitty myself. She, Sayward, and Robin trained me carefully (I did panic just a bit when I saw the size of the syringes involved), and I took copious notes.

I foresee a lot of urine in my future ... but for the moment I also foresee a live cat.

I have no idea which of her lives Lorelei Lee is currently living. Apparently, she—like my mother—has more than nine at her disposal.

It is a huge relief to me that she isn't dying right now, however. I know it's just a matter of time. But it's a matter of time for all of us.

Frankly, I wasn't ready to have kitty hospice as well as mother hospice in the house.

I know my situation is much better than that of many others. I have professional and neighborly support with both my mother and my cat. There are only two of them. And Taffy and Lorelei have lived long, happy, healthy lives. It's hard to complain about the possibility of losing either of them.

Nevertheless, I'm glad to be able to watch Lorelei rest under the woodstove for just a little longer.

Tuesday, November 15: Fate Keeps on Happening

The phrase "fate keeps on happening" comes from the fertile pen of one of my favorite authors.

Anita Loos (1888-1981) wrote novels, memoirs, and screenplays. Her masterpiece, *Gentlemen Prefer Blondes* (1925), was dubbed "the Great American Novel (at last!)" by Edith Wharton in a postcard housed at the Morgan Library (which is lucky enough to have the manuscript of *GPB* as well). Wharton, as they say, knew from novels.

I like the book and its author so much that I named my cat after the blonde whom the novel's gentlemen prefer, Lorelei Lee. Both Loreleis have a habit of using their big blue eyes to entrap less beautiful beings into giving them what they want.

In the case of the feline Lorelei the goal is usually food, preferably chicken. The fictitious Lorelei has internalized the materialism of America in the 1920s and therefore goes for the gold, literally.

"[K]issing your hand may make you feel very, very good," she tells her diary, "but a diamond and sapphire bracelet lasts forever."

I don't take all of the original Lorelei Lee's sayings to heart. If I did, I would be richer and more cosmopolitan. Nevertheless, to me, as to her, fate tends to keep on happening.

I try to plan my life from time to time, but in the end that life seems to follow a course laid out for it by *la forza del destino* or the fickle finger of fate or SOMETHING.

I gather there are people who can shape and control the trajectory of their lives. I don't happen to be one of those people.

I was reminded of this character quirk recently when I read *Remembering the Music, Forgetting the Words* by Kate Whouley. Subtitled "Travels with Mom in the Land of Dementia," this book tells the story of the author's struggles to deal with her late mother's Alzheimer's disease.

Mothers and daughters have different relationships. Kate Whouley's bond with her mother was more conflicted than mine with Taffy. One of the joys of her book is the way in which Whouley seems to resolve their differences as the two women let go of memory and learn to live in the present.

As a writer and as a daughter I was moved by Whouley's description of her mother's diagnosis with Alzheimer's disease and her own acceptance of responsibility for her mother's care. In fact, she explains, she divides their joint experience as adults into "before" and "after"—that is, before and after the diagnosis.

My mother's diagnosis, like much of our life together, was less clear cut. Looking back, my brother David and I agree that she must have had some cognitive impairment in 1998, the year in which our father died.

At the time she seemed her usual sharp self. But … she applied for long-term-care insurance that year and was denied coverage because she failed to pass a brief memory test. She told us that she was distracted during the test, and we believed her.

Taffy had never failed a test in her life, and her memory had always been one of her strengths. One believes what one wants to believe, however.

As the years went by we noted little slips. Taffy repeated the same question over and over again. Formerly fiercely independent, she no longer liked to be alone for long. A prolific reader since early childhood, she had trouble finishing books.

By the time she was officially diagnosed with Alzheimer's disease this past spring by a neurologist, Taffy had been on

Alzheimer's medications for several years. And just about everyone knew that she had dementia.

Nevertheless, we never had an "aha" moment, a point at which we said to ourselves that she was suffering from dementia. It dawned on us little by little.

My role as caregiver was similar. I never actually chose to take care of my mother. It just happened.

I stayed in her house in New Jersey for a couple of years (2000-2002) when I had one of my few-ever formal jobs, at the Museum of Television & Radio (now called the Paley Center for Media) in New York.

When I quit the job to have more time for my writing, Taffy seemed to need more and more company. Gradually, we grew into living together permanently. And gradually I discovered her increasing limitations.

First she needed help driving. Later she lost the capacity to cook simple meals for herself or even eat a sandwich left out for her. Eventually, I realized she couldn't pay her bills or be left for any significant period of time. And so on.

It often seemed as though our world was getting smaller and smaller and smaller. At times this sensation of things closing in frustrated me. I remember a rough Sunday morning a little over a year ago. (Since I'm not a morning person mornings are often my roughest times. It's not darkest only just before the dawn. Just after the dawn can stymie me, too.)

After struggling to get us both dressed and ready for church, I arrived for choir rehearsal with Taffy in tow, short on time and shorter on patience. Our minister, Cara, asked if she could help in any way since I was obviously upset. "Get me my life back!" I cried. It was not one of my finer moments, and I'm sure it worried poor Cara.

Over time, however, moments like that have receded. A number of factors account for this relaxation of tension. First, I have help and support with Taffy—from professional caregivers, from friends and neighbors, from family members. (I never hesitate to ask for help!)

Second, although I blush to admit it, I rejoice that Taffy sleeps later in the morning most of the time now so we generally avoid my worst time of day. Writing about her has also helped me put our life together—its downs and its ups—into perspective.

Above all, things are better because, despite Taffy's weakening condition, we have both moved through the frustration to find new strength in ourselves—not strength of body, but strength in our characters and strength in our relationship.

We focus on life's joys as much as we can and in doing so somehow create joy.

I don't honestly know what might have been different had I realized earlier that my mother had dementia. And I have no idea whether I might have approached living with her any more or less gracefully (or competently) had I chosen rather than fallen into doing so. At this point I can't imagine having done anything else.

I may not have learned how to guide my fate, but I HAVE learned that letting fate keep on happening turns life—even life with dementia—into an adventure. My world with my mother may be small, but it is rich.

Coincidentally, Anita Loos was, like my mother, petite, smart, and lively. She was my mother's current age, 93, when she died, although she claimed she was several years younger.

More power to her.

After all, "a girl like I" (to employ another of the original Lorelei Lee's favorite phrases) can be any age she chooses. Fate may keep on happening, but it can't control the way a girl feels in her mind or in her heart.

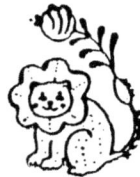

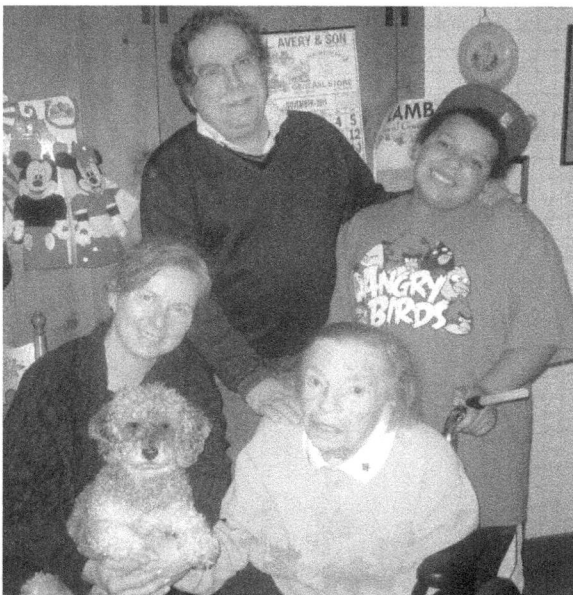

Leigh, David, Michael, and Truffle with Taffy on Thanksgiving

Friday, November 25: A Bountiful Thanksgiving

Thanksgiving is a holiday that speaks of home to most Americans. It also speaks of turkey and cranberry sauce and whatever our personal traditions require at the table, from lasagna to green-bean casserole. But at its heart this holiday is all about home and family.

I've been thinking a lot this year about the meaning of home. Until recently the word "home" came up every day ... sometimes MULTIPLE times per day ... in conversation with my 93-year-old mother.

Like most dementia patients, she pleaded to go home, particularly in the afternoon when the landscape outside darkened.

Taffy's longing for home has often reminded me of Horton Foote's play *The Trip to Bountiful*. Its elderly heroine, Carrie Watts, leads a lonely existence in the house of her uncaring son and daughter-in-law. She longs to return to her childhood home in the now dilapidated town of Bountiful, Texas. To Carrie, Bountiful—I love that name!—represents youth, peace, joy, and love.

We all have our own idealized Bountifuls. I'm lucky that mine is the landscape near my current house in Hawley, Massachusetts. To my late father Bountiful wasn't a physical place. The people he loved constituted his spiritual home.

Years ago my mother told me that her Bountiful was her grandparents' farm in Rutland, Vermont. Her family spent every summer there in her youth.

In her memory Taffy frequently revisited the long, sunny days there, days in which she and her brother wandered the fields, played with friends, or lay on the grass watching clouds drift by. Whatever the real weather may have been, those days were invariably sunny in her recollection.

Lately when Taffy spoke of going home the meaning of the word seemed to shift. Occasionally she was talking about a real house in which she lived as a child with her parents, for she is often a little girl now. As I've written before, I think that home was and is also—and mainly—an archetype to her.

Like Bountiful to Carrie Watts, home to my mother means a figurative place in which she is free of people who don't understand her, free of a body that can no longer do what she asks of it, free of the confusion that besets her mind.

Home may, in fact, mean death to Taffy.

In the last couple of weeks she has asked to go home less frequently. She is weak physically and is getting weaker mentally as well. Wanting to go home takes focus and effort that she doesn't always have anymore. Part of me is relieved: I hated seeing her distressed when she begged to go home. Part of me worries about what comes next.

Every few days she still manages to bleat out a request to go home. When she does I remind her that home is a place in which one is loved. So, I explain, like Dorothy in the film version of *The Wizard of Oz*, she hasn't ever really left home at all.

This explanation generally calms her down. "I am home," she tells me. And we hold hands and smile at each other.

Now, that's something to be thankful for.

Wednesday, November 30: A Bountiful Thanksgiving, Part the Second

I was so busy musing last week about home and Thanksgiving that I forgot to report in on Taffy's literal (as opposed to figurative!) Thanksgiving.

My brother David, his wife Leigh, and their son Michael flew up from Virginia for the holiday weekend. I wouldn't say that my mother could have named them if you had asked her who they were. She was obviously happy to be with them, however.

For the previous couple of weeks she had been sleeping more and more. Even when awake she had kept her eyes closed much of the time, which made getting food into her difficult.

Suddenly on Thanksgiving morning she was alert—watching the Thanksgiving Day parade on television and keeping an eye on the family. She didn't eat a lot of dinner, but she sat at the table with us all and smiled from time to time.

By Friday she was actually beginning to eat ... and she has been eating turkey leftovers ever since. I hope this trend will continue tonight with some other kind of food; we are now officially out of turkey! Happily, we still have pumpkin pie and just a little cranberry-swirl ice cream.

Taffy didn't converse with the family much over the weekend, but she loved the hugs and comfort David and the gang offered.

When they left on Sunday, she was tired ... but the small renaissance begun by their visit has persisted.

Yesterday Taffy was extremely perky. She chatted and laughed. She ate well. She even took a small walk with her walker. (She has been pretty much wheelchair bound for a while.)

Today she is a little more somnolent but by and large still expresses hunger and happiness from time to time. "We have a sassy Taffy today," her caregiver Pam said at lunch.

Jean, the hospice social worker, visited and warned us that this upward trend may not continue. In fact, she explained, weak people often have a spike of good health just before their final decline.

I'm an optimist. I won't exactly ignore Jean's words. She may be right.

I am hopeful, however. And I am thankful for any good days Taffy has. It's heartening to see her personality shine again for a bit.

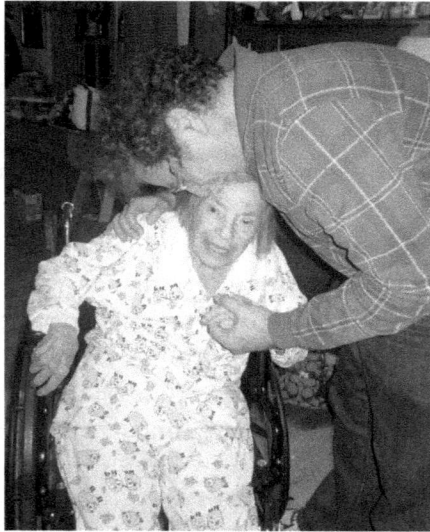

A tired but happy Taffy says goodnight to her firstborn after a very busy Thanksgiving.

November Meditation:
A Smidgen of Advice for Other Caregivers

When I decided to transform my journal entries about my mother into a book, I asked readers of my blog what they thought the book should include in addition to my day-to-day adventures with Taffy.

Several of them suggested that I include some practical tips, things I had learned as a caregiver. In all honesty I have to admit that others suggested I NOT include any advice; they thought that plenty of other books out there fulfilled this function.

(My favorite of these, by the way, is *The Alzheimer's Caregiving Puzzle* [2010] by Patricia R. Callone and Connie Kudlacek.)

I am compromising by including this brief essay, which I hope will make readers facing Alzheimer's disease feel a little less at sea.

My first piece of advice—and I promise you that this is NOT a cop out—is that everyone's experience of living with and dealing with dementia is different and that people's differences should be noted and accepted.

It's true that my family chose to keep my mother at home. ("Chose" may be the wrong word since we more or less fell into it!) This doesn't mean that I think home care is the only route for dealing with the disease.

Things fell into place for us in a lot of ways. I was available and could cut back on my work in order to care for my mother. My mother and I had always gotten along fairly well so we could face living together. Her dementia never got violent, and she was only truly angry and "demented" when suffering from an infection.

She had that rare thing in this day and age, a pension. It enabled us to hire a geriatric adviser to help us plan her path—and home health aides to make my burden lighter. We also had terrific support from our family and our community.

Even so, my brother and I had a back-up plan in place, an assisted-living facility that was willing to take her and care for her if I became ill or just too tired, or if medical advisers came to believe that that care would be better for her.

I have friends who have gone a different route, placing parents (even a spouse in one case) in a care facility.

When making decisions about the best care, I'd say keep these factors in mind:

First, plan ahead so you won't have to make sudden decisions without thinking them through. The back-up plan my brother and I put in place made us much more comfortable with keeping my mother at home.

Second, study your job as caregiver (and it IS a job, even if most of us don't get paid for it!). Learn as much as you can about the disease you face. Talk to your loved one's doctor as much as you can without hurting the patient's feelings. Be willing to try new pharmacological solutions (my mother was wearing an Exelon patch at the end of her life and taking twice-daily doses of Namenda), but watch the patient carefully to make sure that they are working. Ask questions all the time.

Listen to your loved one's words and watch his/her body to try to figure out what you can do to make life better. (People with dementia can't always articulate what they need, but they do give us nonverbal cues.) And listen to your own thoughts and physical symptoms as a caregiver. If you calm down and think things through, you will be able to figure out what path to take. If you are true to your loved one and to yourself, ANY decision you make will be a good decision.

Don't be afraid to reach out and ask for help. Your doctor; county, state, and federal officials; people at places of worship; family members, friends, and neighbors can all help to greater or lesser degrees if you ask them … and if you think hard and try to be specific about the help you need. Sometimes you just need someone to talk to. Find that person. Share your burdens and your joys.

If you think you have come to the end of your tether, wait a few minutes. Life and people's attitudes toward it (especially if those people have dementia!) can change in a very short period of time.

Seek out activities that can make your life and the life of your loved one fuller and more joyful; a little joy can go a long way. In our case, as I have written over and over again, music, fresh air, pets, and laughter were lifesavers again and again. In my case (my mother wasn't strong enough to do much of this) exercise—walking or swimming—also kept my body and mind strong.

Remember that you are in a strange, unique place in life, and so is the person for whom you care. This place can be maddening and challenging. It can also be fun in a crazy way, and it can put you in touch with emotions you didn't know you had. When you look back on it later as I am looking back now, you will realize that all the gifts you have given to your loved one in this place and time have rebounded to you.

November Recipe: Cranberry Swirl Ice Cream

This is one of the last treats Taffy enjoyed; we made it over Thanksgiving weekend.

Ingredients:

for the ice cream:

1-1/2 cups milk

4 egg yolks

2/3 cup sugar

1-1/2 cups heavy cream

2 teaspoons vanilla

1 pinch salt

for the cranberry swirl:

1 cup water

1 cup sugar

12 ounces (3 cups) cranberries

Instructions:

First, make your ice-cream base. Heat the milk until it is steamy but not boiling. In a separate bowl, whisk together the egg yolks and sugar until the mixture is thick and light yellow (about 4 minutes).

Whisk a bit of the hot milk into the egg mixture. Then whisk in more milk, up to about 1/2 or 3/4 cup. Whisk the milky egg yolks into the remaining milk.

Cook over medium heat until the custard begins to thicken but does not boil (about 2 to 3 minutes on my gas stove).

Remove the custard from the heat, and strain it into a heatproof bowl or pot. Cool thoroughly.

As the custard starts to cool make the cranberry sauce to swirl. (It's basically jellied cranberry sauce, but avoid using the canned stuff if possible.)

In a medium saucepan combine the water and sugar and bring them to a boil. Add the cranberries, and return the mixture to a boil. Reduce the heat, and simmer the sauce for 10 more minutes. (If it gets too fuzzy, add a tiny bit of butter.)

Remove the sauce from the heat, and push it through a stainless-steel strainer. You'll end up with about 1-1/2 cups of sauce and a small amount of solid matter; you may discard the latter.

Cool the sauce, covered, at room temperature; then refrigerate it until you are ready to make the ice cream.

When that time comes, use a mixer or whisk to break up the jellied cranberry sauce into a thick liquid (instead of a solid). Measure out 1 cup. You may reserve the rest to put on top of your ice cream if you want extra cranberry flavor.

Go back to your ice-cream base and whisk in the cream, vanilla, and salt. Place this mixture in your ice-cream freezer and begin the churning process.

When the ice cream looks about ready, slowly add the cup of cranberry sauce and continue churning just until you have a pleasing swirled effect. Serve immediately.

This recipe makes a little more than a quart of ice cream.

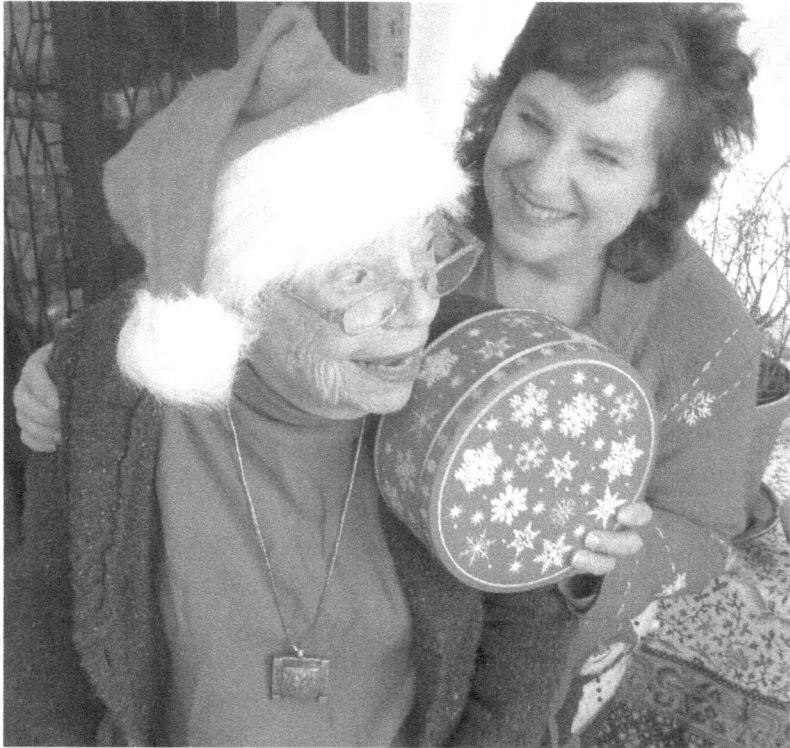

Taffy and Tinky during a previous holiday season

DECEMBER
I'll Fly Away

Monday, December 5: Moral Superiority

Taffy has always been short, although lately she has reached an adult low. She is now about 55 or 56 inches tall. In her prime she got up to 61 and a half inches. This may seem short, but I'm still waiting for a little growth spurt to get me that far!

When my brother grew taller than she was (it didn't take him very long) Taffy looked him in the eye and informed him that she still had "moral superiority." This amorphous term was supposed to mean that he should bow down before her golden character and do her bidding.

In practical terms, it meant that he should do her bidding because her character was extraordinarily forceful. She called herself "strong willed." When the young Tinky exhibited similar characteristics I was told that I was "stubborn." I agree that "strong willed" sounds a lot better.

Taffy inherited many things from her father—her soft brown hair, her square build, her love of literature. Perhaps the most obvious characteristic he bequeathed to her was his legendary and intimidating dead certainty that whatever he said or believed was right.

Having read Oliver Wendell Holmes, my mother called her father "the Autocrat of the Breakfast Table." He always reminded me of Clarence Day Sr. in the book, play, and film *Life with Father*. Like Day, he was a beloved family tyrant.

From my grandfather Taffy absorbed her way of looking a person squarely in the eye and insisting that her opinion equaled the truth no matter what. She has seldom been amenable to argument.

In recent weeks she has retained little energy to assert her opinions and her character. Her method of argument is simply to close her eyes and her mouth and act as though the person who wants to convince her of something (or, often, who wants to feed her a pill) doesn't exist.

This tactic can be frustrating. On the other hand, we caregivers all realize that it is precisely my mother's strength of character that has kept her going as her body has grown weaker and weaker.

So we respect her moments of "moral superiority" and bide our time until her eyes and mouth open again. They seldom remain shut for long. She is too interested in the sights and tastes around her.

Friday, December 9: The Sun Countess

Feminists have long maintained that the separation between public and private (like that between the personal and the political) is basically specious.

My mother was a little older than most of the postwar feminist generation and never called herself a feminist *per se*. Nevertheless, she has gone through life in certainty of the rights and worth of her fellow women.

And she has always viewed public and private behavior as interchangeable. She has lived her life as though every private choice were visible to everyone and every public issue affected her family. She taught me by example to do the same, although I don't always succeed as well as she.

In light of her views on the public/private "split," I think that if she were more lucid Taffy would be pleased with the course of her illness in recent months. And she would be pleased with the way in which she is dying.

She IS dying at this point, I am sad to report. She caught a cold last weekend. The resultant fever has made her weaker and less responsive each day. She barely sips a little broth for nourishment. And she is now completely bedridden. We tried moving her to the living room to sit up yesterday, but she was so stiff and weak that we decided not to try taking her out of her bed again unless she gets better. This seems unlikely.

Despite being in bed and being minimally conscious, she still receives her public. She's not quite the Sun King, Louis XIV, who was rumored to have a hundred courtiers in attendance each morning when he arose and dressed.

I'm dubbing her the Sun Countess, with enough attendants and visitors to evoke an occasional smile and to keep her comfortable.

Hospice sends nurses and aides. We have our faithful helpers Pam and Jen. My brother is around, and Taffy always seems to respond a little to his touch. Friends and neighbors call and stop by to say hello.

I'm proud that in recent months we have taken her out into the sunshine and the larger world as often as we could. And I'm happy that that world is wishing her well as her journey nears its end. Every life and every death need to be public as well as private.

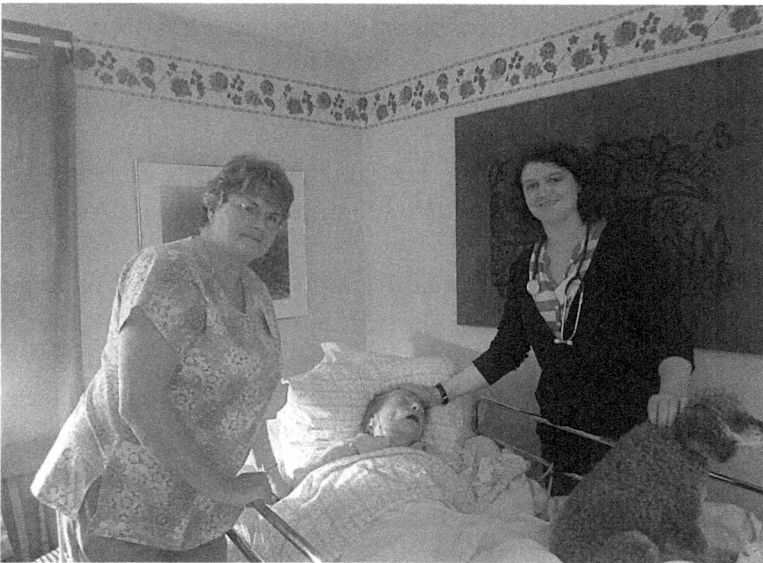

Jackie (left) and Sarah from Hospice of Franklin County check on Taffy.

Tuesday, December 13: I'll Fly Away

Taffy died a little after 9:30 on Sunday night. Jennifer, one of her dear aides, was by her side. I had left the room for a couple of minutes to write an email. My little mother was sleeping peacefully and just stopped breathing.

We had a weekend surrounded by family and friends who gave both of us comfort. My brother had to leave Sunday morning to return to his family in Virginia, but he spent much of the weekend with our mother, who always responded just a little to her firstborn.

Sunday was tricky for Taffy. For much of the day she seemed to be struggling to speak, to train her brain on some important matter, to make her body do what it could no longer do. We told her that we loved her and played and sang Christmas carols. Eventually, she grew calm and drifted off.

Our faithful dog Truffle lay quietly by Taffy's side for many hours that day, sensing that climbing up to kiss her was no longer feasible.

Just after Taffy died I brought Truffle in to say goodbye. She no longer wanted to jump onto the bed. She seemed to know that the body lying there no longer held her mother.

Originally my dog, Truffle became more and more my mother's pet in the past couple of years, a bond I welcomed for both their sakes. Yesterday Truffle was a little bewildered but soon established herself as mine once more, sticking close to me and to the cat.

Taffy gave me many gifts over the years. Unwittingly she shared one last gift. About a month ago I used her money to order myself a red flannel nightgown. She was beyond shopping, but I was sure she would want to give me a Christmas present.

When she became bedridden the hospice aides suggested that a nightgown would be easier to maneuver in the bed than her usual pajamas. Unfortunately, Taffy had no cold-weather nighties.

I went upstairs and took the red flannel gown out of its wrappings. She was wearing it when she died. I'll think of her generosity of spirit every time I put it on.

I have been flooded with phone calls and messages, which have touched me deeply. Here is the obituary we sent to newspapers.

Jan Weisblat

Jan Hallett Weisblat, 93, of Hawley, Massachusetts, and Alexandria, Virginia, died at her home in Massachusetts on Sunday, December 11, 2011. She also considered Millburn, New Jersey, her home; she lived there from 1972 to 2010.

Janice Elizabeth Hallett was born on September 26, 1918, in Brooklyn, New York, the child of Erwin Bruce Hallett, an attorney, and Clara Engel Hallett, a homemaker. Her family moved to New Jersey when she was very small. She spent her life dividing her time between New Jersey and New England, with forays overseas.

She graduated *cum laude* from Mount Holyoke College in 1939 with a major in French and studied education at the Bank Street School. She later received a master's degree in French from Seton Hall University. She taught elementary school, secondary school, and even college over the years. She loved teaching, learning, and young people.

After saying yes to numerous proposals but never accepting a ring from any of the young men involved, Jan Hallett took a ring from Abe Weisblat, whom she met while both were teaching at Stevens Hoboken Academy in Hoboken, New Jersey.

The bride was Christian and the groom Jewish so their parents asked them to remain engaged for at least a year before marrying in order to be sure that the "mixed" marriage would take. It took and lasted from 1945 until Abe Weisblat's death in 1998.

Over the course of their marriage the pair lived in India, the Philippines, and Great Britain as well as the United States. Jan Weisblat had special love for India and France. She wrote a book of poems called "My India" and was frequently taken for French by native speakers of that language.

In 1958 her family first visited Singing Brook Farm in Hawley, Massachusetts. The Weisblats spent every summer at the Farm from then on, eventually building a year-round house in Hawley. Abe Weisblat called it "Ashram West." His wife called it home.

She loved history and old things. In the 1970s she and her friend Claire Roth started an antique shop in Charlemont, Massachusetts, the Charlemont House Gallery. When her partner retired, Weisblat moved the shop to nearby Shelburne Falls and christened it the Merry Lion in honor of her *alma mater*'s founder, Mary Lyon.

She ran her store with the help of the late folk artist Judith Russell, who often painted the view of the Bridge of Flowers from the shop window. The Merry Lion specialized in Staffordshire plates, pressed glass, and whimsy. Its proprietress retired in 2001 to enjoy being a grandmother (at last!).

An avid amateur thespian, she loved to recite poetry, particularly nonsense verse like "The Owl and the Pussycat" and "The Pobble Who Has No Toes." She was a loyal friend and wife, a demanding but loving mother, and a generous no-fuss hostess. Bright and funny, she loved crossword puzzles, music, and good conversation.

Decades after her graduation from Mount Holyoke a professor was asked whether he recalled Janice Hallett. "Short and full of life!" he responded, providing her epitaph.

She is survived by her two siblings, Bruce Hallett of Manchester Center, Vermont, and Lura Hallett Smith of Southbury, Connecticut. She also left a son, David Weisblat, of Alexandria, Virginia, along with his wife Leigh and their son Michael; a daughter, Tinky Weisblat, of Hawley, Massachusetts; and numerous nieces and nephews.

A brief memorial service will be held at the Federated Church in Charlemont, Massachusetts, on Saturday, January 7, at 1 p.m. A larger celebration is being planned for the spring.

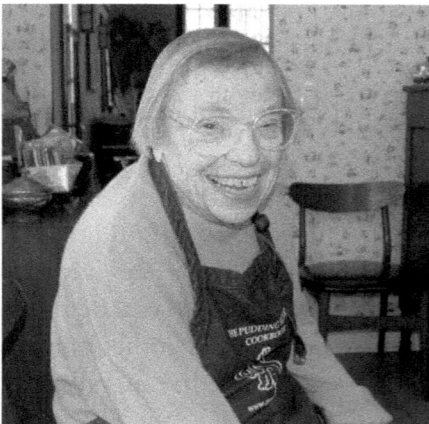

Our dear friend Judy Christian took this picture of a smiling Taffy.

Thursday, December 29: Looking Back

When I began this year-long project of writing about my mother I had no idea that fate was planning to provide closure for us with my mother's death in December. A few days after my mother passed away, as if to reinforce the truth that my life and my story were changing, I had to say goodbye to our cat, Lorelei Lee.

Both died quietly and gently after long, happy lives. Both died surrounded by love. A girl can get a little sick of the words "it was very peaceful." There are worse ways to die, however, and worse ways to lose loved ones.

A few days ago I sat down to read all that I have written to date here. Looking back, I am pleased with what this project has helped me accomplish this year.

It enabled me to cope—more than cope—with my mother's illness. The first few essays seemed to dwell an awful lot on the difficulties of taking care of her. As the year went on, however, I became more attuned to the pluses of caregiving and less upset by the minuses. Tears of frustration turned into tears of tenderness.

I began by writing about what I was losing. Somewhere along the line I started writing about what I was finding. In short, a burden was transformed into a privilege.

I recently discovered the blog *Momma and Me*. Its author, Arlene, lives in Texas and takes care of her mother, who has Lewy Body Dementia. Arlene isn't a professional writer, but her words about her mother shine with love.

In her very first post, written in March 2011, Arlene wrote about having to install locks and an alarm on her door in an attempt to keep her Momma from wandering off. "I'm locking the door, but not my heart," she wrote.

Arlene knew right away what it has taken me a year—actually a lifetime—to learn. My resolution for the coming new year is that I will never lock my heart.

In addition to teaching me about love and caregiving, *Pulling Taffy* has made friends for me as I put portions of it onto the internet in blog form. It has also enabled friends and relatives I haven't been able to see much to reach out to me. I am grateful for this companionship.

Miraculously, in writing these essays I have become a better writer, a better daughter, and (I hope) a better person.

I'm not sure what the year to come holds for my little dog and me. The days since my mother's death have been full of activity and affection. Concerned about my newly orphaned status, my friends and family have showered me with cards, emails, gifts, food, phone calls, favors, memories, and good times.

Christmas was a magical day of family and feasting. My tiny tree (obtained and decorated with my nephew Michael on Christmas Eve) gleams in my sun room. Almost every ornament in the collection I inherited from Taffy represents a happy time we had together. My family has recalled my father this season as well, both in stories and in lighting the Chanukah menorah.

I know that things will quiet down and that I will have sad moments. Our poor little dog Truffle is frequently sad these days, staying as close as she can to the family she has left. I know that she and I will survive these moments with humor, music, friendship, long walks, and lots of belly rubs. (The last two are officially for Truffle but will probably help me as well.)

As I look ahead I believe that the best way to honor my mother's memory and to keep myself stable is to emulate her and be as useful as I can be. And above all to cultivate the joy she felt almost every day. I don't have her smile, but I'll make good use of my own.

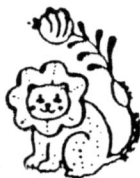

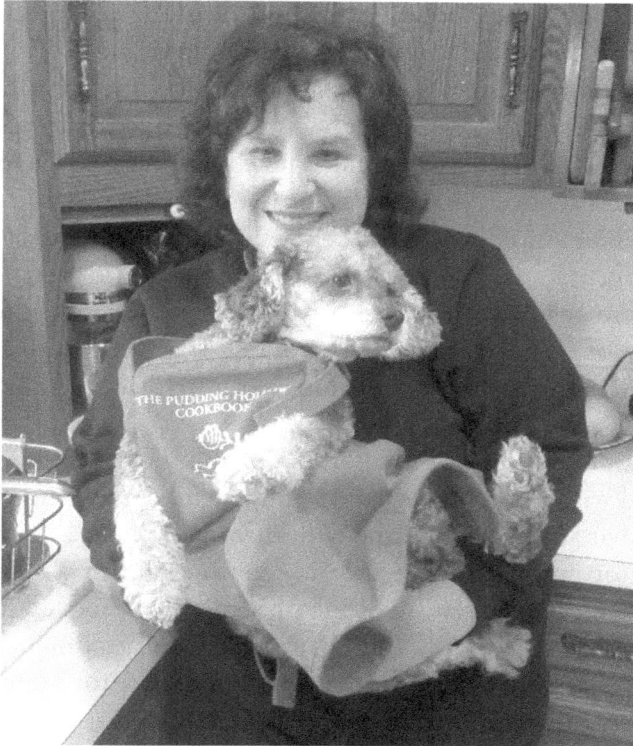

And then there were two.....

December Meditation: Pushing Tinky

This book has been about my mother and our relationship. Relationships aren't over when a person's life is over, however, and in any case I thought readers might like to find out how I have fared since Taffy's death.

Grief manifests itself differently in different people. I miss my mother—and I weep for her from time to time, mostly when I'm short on sleep. Late one night a few months after her death I was wandering around in a daze and broke one of her wineglasses. It wasn't her favorite wine glass or one of her most valuable pieces of crystal, but suddenly I felt like a terrible daughter and started crying. After a while, I recalled Taffy's dislike of tears and her practicality. And I got over my crying jag.

In general my thoughts about my mother are more positive than they were that night. She is never far from my thoughts, even when I am at work. She still seems to sing along as I practice my music. And she would enjoy my writing projects.

When someone dies the strangest thing—to me, at any rate—is how "not there" he or she suddenly is. Where once there was color we are left with black and white. Where once there was a voice we are left with silence. Memories color in the shadows and make the voice audible once again. And fellowship reminds us that we are never alone.

I try to stay busy, although I will never manage to be as busy as Taffy was in her prime; she was the ultimate multitasker. I do my best to view both my time alone and my financial situation as challenges rather than disadvantages.

The time alone is easy to fill. I still inhabit the rich communities I enjoyed with Taffy. Friends and family members continue to visit and to invite me to spend time with them.

One of my first moves after my mother's death was to get a new kitten, the irrepressible Rhubarb (Ruby for short). Although she cuts into my sleep with her inclination to play all night and all day, Ruby has been a tonic for me—and even more for Truffle, who desperately needed someone else to love. They are firm friends, and Truffle and I are seldom bored. The act of naming the cat alone entertained my family, my friends, and me for several weeks.

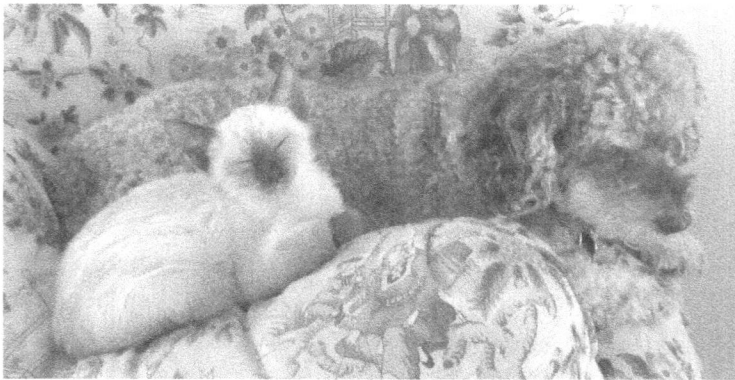

I try to stay true to Taffy by keeping in touch with her brother and sister. Talking to them and being with them is a pleasure as well as a duty.

So my social life is rich. My finances are more of a challenge.

I get lots of literature from our local hospice group about dealing with grief, but nothing I've read talks about the financial side of loss. It seems somehow less than dignified to think about money when you are grieving—but then dignity has never been my strong suit.

Income has never been my strong suit, either.

I laugh when politicians describe education as the key to good jobs and incomes. People don't come a lot more educated than I. I have an A.B. degree (no mere B.A. for me, thank you very much) in French and astronomy, a master's degree in journalism, and a Ph.D. in American studies. I have written three theses, and I have been elected into numerous scholastic honor societies.

I also have certificates from two legendary but now defunct institutions. I took a secretarial course at the Katharine Gibbs School after college to learn shorthand and typing. And somewhere in the files I ought to be able to lay my hands on my diploma from London's Lucie Clayton Finishing School. There I learned such useful skills as how to get in and out of a sports car without separating my knees and how to shake hands with the queen.

Despite all my diplomas and academic honors I have never made much money.

To some extent my inability to generate income is a legacy from my parents. They always maintained that income didn't matter, that work should be fulfilling rather than remunerative.

To a greater extent, of course, my lack of salary is my own darn fault. The few times that I have worked in offices I have felt stifled. I actually like to work; I just don't want to work during the exact same hours in the exact same location every day.

As a result I have concentrated on my writing, which has given me great joy but little money.

The next year or two will be a grand experiment for me. I have enough savings to last for a while as I reinvent myself.

Some of those funds came from my parents' art collection. About nine months after my mother's death my brother David and I sold a number of paintings at Sotheby's auction house in New York to create an additional financial cushion.

The art was collected over a 20-year period (roughly 1960 to 1980) and is primarily from India. Our parents had no formal training in art, but they had a strong feeling for color, composition, and the creative process.

It was hard to say goodbye to many of the bright canvasses that had adorned our walls for many years. We are keeping quite a number of pieces, however, so the walls won't be entirely bare. And working on the essay about our parents for the Sotheby's sale catalogue prompted David, his wife Leigh, and me to go through a treasure trove of old letters, diaries, and photographs. (I used some of them for my meditations in this book!)

Looking through these documents has taught us a lot. We may be losing art, but we have gained priceless perspective on our parents' marriage and on their attitudes toward the world and each other. Seeing their lives as a whole in retrospect like this, we have been struck again and again by their courage, their strength, their practicality, their commitment to social justice, and their likability.

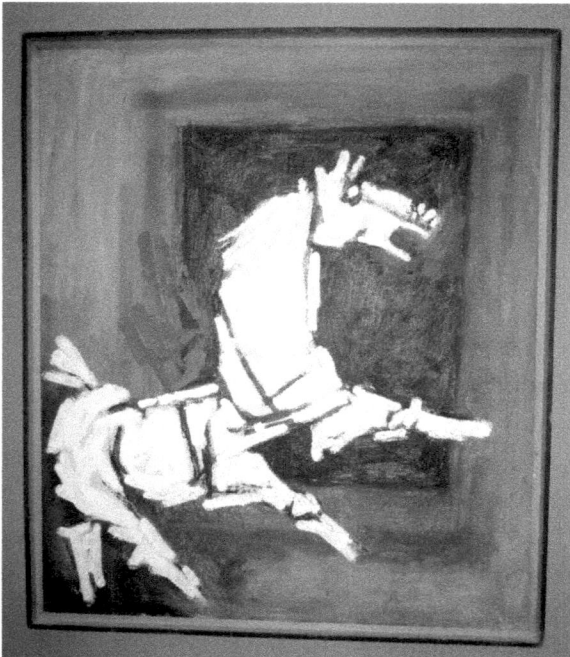

This lovely horse still graces my living room.

They amassed their art collection in large part because they provided a welcoming home for some of their artist friends' favorite paintings. Our largest painting ended up on their living-room wall simply because its creator had a fondness for it and didn't want to sell it to anyone else.

I have just realized that I used the word "home" AGAIN in the last paragraph. At Taffy's memorial service our friend and neighbor Alice described Taffy as a homemaker. I had never used that word to describe her, but as I look back at her life, and particularly at the year chronicled in this book, the word "home" inescapably crops up over and over again.

One use of the word appears in my descriptions of Taffy's recurring desire to go "home." That one word encompassed many meanings to her and to me. It was seldom far from her lips during that year.

She also had a remarkable ability to create home and community wherever she was. She started out thinking of New Jersey as home, and it certainly continued to represent stable happiness for her throughout her life. Nevertheless, as these pages have attested, she found and made homes in Rutland, Vermont; in South Hadley, Massachusetts, at Mount Holyoke; in Paris, France; and in Bombay and New Delhi, India.

Other places represented home to her over the years as well— Washington, D.C., where she and my father spent their first few years of married life; London, England, where Taffy home schooled me for a few months; and Madison, Wisconsin, where she taught school and held a salon in their apartment while my father did graduate work.

She was at home in the kitchen and in the world of literature. She was at home speaking French or English; she even dabbled confidently in Spanish, Italian, Tagalog, and Hindi. She was at home in the theater and in the concert hall. She was at home arguing with adults or playing with children.

In short, she was at home in the world. As I look toward my future, I know that thanks to her example I will never be without a moral compass, a community of friends and relatives, or a home.

December Recipe: Salt-Water Taffy

I couldn't end this book without a recipe for taffy! I wouldn't call this easy to make. You need to have quick, strong pullers. (Four to six would be the ideal number.) Nevertheless, it's worth a try. I'm still working on my pulling skills: my most recent batch was a little TOO chewy. But the flavor made it well worth chewing.

Ingredients:

2 cups sugar
1 cup light corn syrup
1 cup water
1-1/2 teaspoons salt
2 tablespoons sweet butter at room temperature, plus additional butter later for hands
1 generous splash vanilla

Instructions:

Butter a large jelly-roll pan (or 2 small ones). Better yet, place a silicone mat on the pan or pans—and butter that as well!

In a heavy, 3-quart saucepan over medium heat, combine the sugar, corn syrup, water, and salt. Bring the mixture to a boil, stirring until the sugar dissolves. Place a candy thermometer in the side of the pan and continue to cook, without stirring, until the mixture reaches 260 degrees (the hard-ball stage). Be careful: the temperature tends to rise slowly at first and then escalate! I never trust my candy thermometer entirely so I keep a small dish of cold water nearby and test the candy BEFORE I think it might be ready by dripping a little into the dish to see whether I have a hard ball.

Remove the mixture from the heat, and stir in the butter and vanilla. Carefully pour the molten candy onto the prepared pan or pans. Let it stand until you can JUST handle it

Quickly divide the candy into halves, then into additional sections depending on how many pullers you have. With buttered hands pull the taffy rapidly and energetically until it turns white and begins to be difficult to pull. Twist the taffy into ropes, and snip them into 1-inch pieces with buttered scissors or a serrated knife. Wrap the pieces in wax paper. You should have 60 to 75 pieces of candy.

Acknowledgments

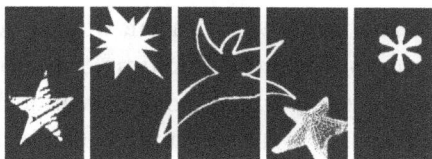

I have so many people to thank for their help with this book (and during the year in which it takes place) that I have a feeling I'm doomed to forget someone, like the queen in a fairy tale who can't remember to invite everyone to her child's Christening. If I have inadvertently omitted you, please do not claim my firstborn child!

First, I want to thank my immediate family—David, Leigh, and Michael—for their help with this book and for their support in everything I do. They have helped organize files, move furniture, and taste weird food. They make my life richer every day. Leigh in particular stepped in to help with proofreading and recipe testing when both seemed to be getting the better of me.

Blessings on the brave folks who agreed to look at this manuscript in its first draft: Paul Ashdown, R. Peter Beck, Margot Bullard, and Horace Newcomb. All made suggestions that helped to shape the final book. If I didn't implement them all properly, the fault is entirely mine. And Peter not only provided counsel (and treats!) over the years but also came up with the title "Pulling Taffy." He took the cover photo for this book as well.

I am grateful to Leslie Fields at the Mount Holyoke College archives for hunting down the poem "You, In Proud White Dress"—and to Lisa Johnson for sharing publishing advice.

Thanks to the passionate readers of my blog. Some of you I knew before I began this journey. Many I did not. You gave me advice, support, and comfort.

Thanks to the wonderful professional caregivers who helped with my mother—Pam Gerry, Jennifer Rich, Joan Sutton, Joan De Gusto, Mitch Opalski, Pertina Wallace, and Brenda Walker. I would never have had time to think, let alone write, had it not been for you. You showed me what it means to do a job with love.

And thanks to the helpful people at Hospice of Franklin County. Our team members (Jackie Baker, Jean Footit, Dvora Cohen, and Rose Kiablick) were crucial, but we received counsel from just about everyone there at one time or another.

I also wish to express gratitude for my wonderful community. Here I mention just a few among many. David and Sally Rich brought us water during the hurricane, Cara Hochhalter visited weekly, Will Cosby and Lisa Johnson stopped by whenever they could, the Gillans brought cheer and food, Betsy Kovacs and Jack Estes helped rearrange the house for an invalid, Mary Stuart and Ellen Cosby shared counsel and trash facilities, and Esther Haskell understood when I didn't show up to sing in choir because of a maternal crisis. The caring staff at Avery's Store bodily lifted Taffy into the building to shop and always greeted her with a smile.

Above all, Alice Parker Pyle came to see us every day when she was in town, always drawing a smile from my mother. She sat vigil with me the day my mother died and helped in a hundred other small and large ways, basically defining the term "good neighbor."

Thanks to the Charlemont-Hawley Cultural Council for helping to fund my work on *Pulling Taffy*. The money was of course useful—but the recognition and vote of confidence were even more of a boon.

I dedicate this book to the memory of my parents. I hope I grow up to be as wise, brave, and funny as they were.

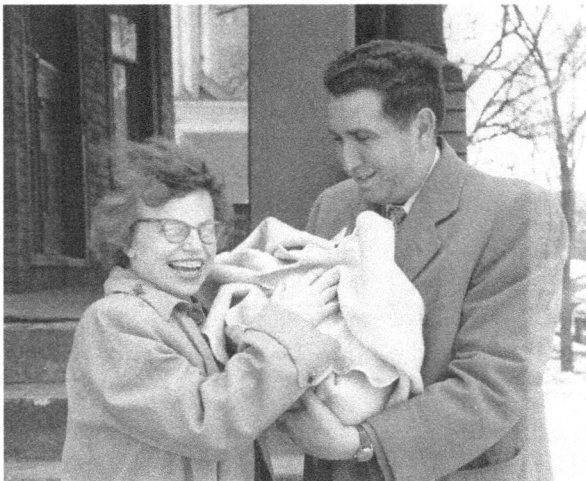

With Baby David in April 1953

www.ingramcontent.com/pod-product-compliance
Lightning Source LLC
Chambersburg PA
CBHW052040090426
42739CB00010B/1991